Urgent care handbook

Professional practice

Note

Healthcare practice and knowledge are constantly changing and developing as new research and treatments, changes in procedures, drugs and equipment become available.

The author and publishers have, as far as is possible, taken care to confirm that the information complies with the latest standards of practice and legislation.

Urgent care handbook
Professional practice

by

Lynda Sibson

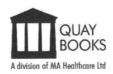

QUAY
BOOKS

A division of MA Healthcare Ltd

Quay Books Division, MA Healthcare Ltd, St Jude's Church, Dulwich Road, London SE24 0PB

British Library Cataloguing-in-Publication Data
A catalogue record is available for this book

© MA Healthcare Limited 2010

ISBN-10: 1-85642-406-5
ISBN-13: 978-1-85642-406-6

Printed by CLE, Huntingdon, Cambridgeshire

Contents

Preface

This book is aimed at advanced healthcare professionals working in urgent and pre-hospital care settings in the UK in the following clinical areas: the pre-hospital setting, primary care, community clinics, emergency departments, walk-in centres, urgent care clinics, minor injury clinics and out-of-hours clinics. There will undoubtedly be other facilities and organisations providing care in the urgent setting; any omission is entirely mine and I apologise in advance.

The book is predominantly, although not exclusively, aimed at practitioners working as paramedics and nurses in the clinical areas identified above. These practitioners will be qualified and registered with the Health Professions Council or the Nursing and Midwifery Council and possess considerable clinical expertise. They could be nurse practitioners, emergency nurse practitioners, paramedics, advanced clinical practitioners, paramedic practitioners, consultant nurses, paramedics, and so on. However, it is important to stress that the book should be useful to all healthcare professionals at any stage in their career and irrespective of their title role or the setting in which they work.

I would urge you to read the chapters that do not reflect your professional group. The rationale for this is to encourage you to understand how the other professional groups practice and how they have developed. There are some distinct similarities and many potential opportunities for shared practice.

Section One focuses on the professional and educational development of paramedics and nurses. *Chapter 1* focuses on some of the historical developments underpinning the paramedic role with an outline of the policy and professional issues that have been associated with the development of the extended and advanced paramedic roles. The chapter also outlines the development of some of the specialist roles that have developed within the paramedic profession. *Chapter 2* is concerned with nursing practice, exploring the history and background to the developing and evolving roles of nurses.

Section Two refers to clinical leadership in clinical practice and its potential role in supporting practitioners in their professional role. Clinical leadership is further explored through the concepts of clinical supervision, mentorship and reflective practice.

Section Three focuses on the key legal and ethical issues in relation to urgent healthcare. The five ethical principles of autonomy, nonmaleficence, beneficence, dignity and justice are discussed, highlighting some key issues relevant to urgent and pre-hospital care.

The Handbook aims to act as a reference guide and to promote and generate discussion. As in all good and progressing practice, feedback and comments are welcome.

Lynda Sibson

Acknowledgements

There are many friends, colleagues, students, patients, academic and teaching staff who have assisted in my nursing career over the years and since this book is really the culmination of all of my experience, learning and teaching, I owe thanks to them all.

Particularly thanks go to the staff at Mark Allen Publishing and Quay Books for providing me with the opportunity to publish what will hopefully be the first of several books. I would like specifically to thank Professor Andy Newton for his experience, knowledge, original humour and contribution to *Chapter 1*, also Sue Hailes for her assistance and insight in *Section Three*. I also wish to thank Hilary Orpet, for inspiration, support, publishing advice and guidance over the years

To Sarah Minster and Suzanne Moss – two wonderful, unique women who are always there for me. I am indebted to you both.

Finally, to my wonderful children, Hannah and Jacob, and my husband Jay, for his everlasting love and support whilst I have embarked on my unique and much loved career in nursing.

Section One

Professional practice

This section focuses on the development of paramedic and nursing practice. As a precursor to pre-hospital care, many nursing and paramedic roles were defined by, and evolved from, military conflict, when care lacked both professional and regulatory guidance.

Paramedic practice developed from the military battlefields with the transport of wounded soldiers to field hospitals for trauma care. There followed an initial patchy adoption in civilian life for the transfer of patients to hospital. The paramedic role today involves a much greater range of care provision within the pre-hospital setting, with great strides having been made in the delivery of clinical care at the scene and en route to hospital. This continues to evolve with the specialisation of the paramedic role into a paramedic practitioner managing patients in the urgent and primary care setting, autonomously, without the need for referral or transfer to hospital. This has often been achieved with the collaboration of other healthcare professionals, such as primary care nurses working in GP surgeries or with district nurses in the community. The preparation for paramedic practice is changing from the traditional didactic training model to a more adult-orientated academic programme of study in a higher educational institute setting. This is in preparation for the development of these roles and to underpin the evolving profession.

The role of the nurse has changed dramatically over the years as the profession has evolved, with many nurses retaining a "general" role in hospital. Others have specialised in community and primary care settings, for example as nurse practitioners and specialist clinical nurses whose work has focused on specific area such as cardiac medicine, respiratory medicine and diabetes. These new roles have required nurses to assume some of the traditional roles of doctors, namely examination of and prescribing for the patient. As the profession grew and the nature of urgent care changed, the need for greater professional requirements emerged. This has also led to the development of professional guidelines and advanced research practices.

CHAPTER I

Paramedic practice

Lynda Sibson and Andy Newton

This chapter focuses on the emergence of the paramedic practitioner role, an emergence that has been in response to new advances in clinical practice and the associated changes in clinical demand. For the paramedic profession, such advances are still relatively new. This chapter also highlights some of the obstacles and barriers that new professions face.

History of paramedic practice

According to Goode (1960) industrialising societies are professionalising societies, and perhaps nowhere is this more apparent than in the rise of the allied health professional (AHP). The UK nursing profession was well established by 1960s and many other AHPs, such as physiotherapists and radiographers, were operating in a form that is recognisable today. However until comparatively recently, the paramedic role was almost non-existent.

Historically, the role was often associated with armed conflict. It was initially evident in the Imperial Legions of Rome, where ageing, non-active centurions were tasked with retrieving and treating wounded soldiers from the battlefields. Some of these centurions would have undertaken crude surgical procedures, such as amputations and suturing wounds, although they would have had little or no training.

The first horse-drawn ambulances, initially intended for rapid retrieval of wounded soldiers, were in civilian use for some 100 years, for example, for recovering the dead during the plague outbreaks in London in 1598 and 1665. It was during the American Civil War that Dr Jonathan Letterman, an American surgeon credited with developing many of the modern methods for military medical organisation, established field hospitals serviced by an efficient ambulance corps with a well-organised medical supplies distribution system. Following the war, some of the veterans began replicating this system in their civilian communities, with volunteer life-saving teams and ambulance corps.

In post-war UK, early ambulance services were operated by hospitals or the police services. In some larger cities they were often run by a combination of the police, fire service and the local health department. During the First World War, motorised ambulances were successfully trialed on the battlefield and were subsequently utilised in the civilian setting. The actual date of the beginning of the role of the first paramedic, or "ambulance attendant" as they were known, is unclear, but the consensus points to the US in 1928 in Roanoke, Virginia when Julian Wise helplessly witnessed two men drowning. Unable to save the men by himself, Wise vowed never to have to observe such an event again and formed a volunteer rescue squad.

As time progressed, clinical skills advanced and it was during the Second World War that battlefield "medics" first administered opiate analgesia whilst performing emergency procedures. During the Korean War, helicopters were widely utilised for the medical evacuation of the wounded to medical units, the first "medevac" patients, although this form of transportation did not enter civilian life for another 20 years.

Today, the paramedic title is protected by law, with all paramedics being required to undertake a programme of study that has been recognised and validated by the Health Professions Council. Paramedics usually work as part of the emergency medical service either in a land or air ambulance providing emergency on-scene pre-hospital care to a range of patients in a variety of settings.

Development of the UK ambulance service

The modern ambulance service developed following the 1946 National Health Services Act (Department of Health, 1946) when local authorities were required to provide ambulances where necessary. Prior to this, access to an ambulance was a postcode lottery with ambulances being available in cities and large towns, staffed initially by local volunteers who simply transferred patients to hospital, with little or no care provided en route. The Millar Report (Ministry of Health, 1966, 1967) recommended that ambulance crews should receive intensive training in first aid, the management of seriously ill patients, lifting and handling, and driving. Following the Millar Report a number of local training courses were established, including life-saving procedures such as haemorrhage control, neck and back injury care, cardiopulmonary resuscitation and fluid, drug and oxygen therapy. In the mid 1980s the Department of Health requested that the then National Health Service Training Directorate develop a training package for the introduction of ambulance paramedics into the UK ambulance service. This package, as the Millar recommendations, was very much skills-based (Kilner, 2004).

Since this time, the concept of the UK ambulance service has changed radically, evolving at an increasing pace with greater emphasis on clinical treatment rather than the more historical transport function. This trend, beginning in the 1970s when the first paramedics (then termed extended trained ambulance staff) were developed, appears to have increased the ratio of non-life-threatening to life-threatening calls. In parallel, there has been an expansion of the clinical capability of ambulance professionals, particularly in respect to a continued treatment and management focus on patients with immediately life-limiting conditions.

More recently a much greater emphasis has been placed on the recognition of the fundamental change in priorities with patient assessment, treatment and, where necessary, appropriate referral becoming more common, with less demand for resuscitative care and potentially less requirement for transport too. However, changing the role of paramedics in this way, while logical, is a major undertaking and must be accomplished safely. Some early research in the US, such as the "Red River" work in New Mexico and the much larger studies by Bissell et al (1999), raise concerns that the patient assessment skills taught within most paramedic programmes would generally be insufficient to carry out safe and effective field triage.

Changes to pre-hospital medicine affecting paramedic practice

While the paramedic role has been developing, it is worth outlining the simultaneous changes in pre-hospital medicine. Pre-hospital cardiac care was the first to be made available, in Belfast in 1966, where a mobile coronary care unit for defibrillating patients was developed (Geddes, 1986). The initial technology was very basic (a car battery powering a portable defibrillator) compared to the technology being utilised in military and space programmes which was initially deemed too expensive for the pre-hospital care setting in North America, although it was available in Europe and the UK.

Some of the key research being undertaken in the US included the publication by the National Academy of Sciences in 1966 of a landmark paper entitled *Accidental death and disability: The neglected disease of modern society*. This influential document was the result of research into US emergency medical care and it heavily criticised the standard and availability of ambulance equipment and training of attendants, highlighting that soldiers wounded in Vietnam received better care than those injured in road traffic accidents in the US. This led to the improved training of these ambulance attendants, leading to the role of the emergency medical technician.

As a direct result of this report, three US centres began developing pilot paramedic programmes, initially aiming to ensure that fire departments in all major cities would have a team of paramedic-trained fire-fighters. It was through a popular television series, called *Emergency!* that the role became accepted by the public and emergency personnel alike. The show's technical advisor, a senior fire officer named James Page, went on to establish the *Journal of Emergency Medical Services*.

During the 1970s and 1980s, the US ambulance service evolved, with paramedic training delivered locally, to meet communities' needs. This resulted in a wide variety of training and service provision, culminating with

5

the common standard and examination for the role of the emergency medical technician and paramedic seen today.

In the UK, a similar two-tier system of technician and paramedic, the former equated to the US emergency medical technician, existed, with both trained to a common curriculum, originally accredited by the Institute of Health and Care Development (IHCD). The IHCD awards were delivered at two levels: the technician award and the paramedic award, the latter being a longer, more in-depth programme. Individuals would undertake the technician programme, then commence the paramedic programme, if so desired, once they had consolidated their technician training. Many technicians took the logical step of undertaking the IHCD paramedic examination to upgrade.

Development of the paramedic role

In 2000, the Joint Royal Colleges Ambulance Liaison Committee (JRCALC), in partnership with the now disbanded Ambulance Services Association, proposed the development of the expanded role of practitioner in emergency care (Chamberlain, 2000). This new practitioner in emergency care role aimed to broaden the skills and knowledge of paramedics in order to meet the diverse clinical needs of patients, particularly those with undifferentiated but non-life-threatening healthcare issues. The role of the practitioner in emergency care, designed to "up-skill" paramedics, had wide support from the trade unions. At the same time, paramedics joined the ranks of AHPs as the 12th professional group admitted to the AHP Career Framework register.

Increasing demand for pre-hospital health services, specifically unscheduled or urgent care, largely drove the demand for an emergency contact service. Patient demand behaves rather like the flow of water; it follows the line of least resistance. The 999 system is the one NHS service that was designed without an expectation that there would be a need for a "gate-keeping" function, hence its construction without "road blocks". This situation has altered with the advent of triage that is designed to redirect, moderate flow or reject requests; a "traffic light" system. However, controversy continues as to what constitutes "appropriate" demand for ambulance services and few criteria have been developed by which to judge the legitimacy of a 999 call.

Research has identified similar results with regard to "inappropriate" calls to the ambulance service. Palazzo et al (1998) reported rates of 15.7% of "inappropriate" calls to UK ambulance services, the US reported similar results with Schmidt et al (2000) suggesting that 21.3% of ambulance transfers were clinically inappropriate whilst Dunne et al (2003), applying a tighter definition, revealed that 59.2% of ambulance calls were clinically unnecessary, noting that specific training and triage protocols were required to assist paramedic decision making. Such definitions of "inappropriateness" are of course, to some extent, in the eye of the beholding researcher and also affected by the capabilities of the ambulance service. It is arguable that it is this increasing demand for an immediate response from the emergency ambulance service, coupled with a gradual escalating of clinical capability that have driven changes in the role of ambulance paramedics and the creation of new roles, such as that of emergency care assistant.

The objective of reducing this "inappropriate" demand, particularly in terms of unnecessary transportation of patients to emergency departments, is not new. Sir Kenneth Calman, former Chief Medical Officer, addressed some of the key issues in his final report *Developing emergency services in the community* (Department of Health, 1997). To come full circle, in terms of developing the workforce to enable more effective and better co-ordinated care for patients, Professor Chamberlain as then Chair of JRCALC in partnership with the Ambulance Services Association, created the practitioner in emergency care role (JRCALC and Ambulance Services Association, 2000).

The rationale for the development of the practitioner in emergency care role was based on the recognition that not all 999 calls represented hyper-acute emergencies. The vast majority of calls were for less serious "undifferentiated" primary care type issues. The role of the practitioner in emergency care was an initial attempt at workforce development and modernisation, moving towards an ambulance service that could evolve into an effective delivery system of "mobile health care" where the requirements of up to 30% of patients could be met by a higher level paramedic practitioner (JRCALC and Ambulance Services Association, 2000).

The supporting Ambulance Services Association document, *The future of ambulance services in the United Kingdom,* strongly supported the idea that ambulance services should move from "bringing patients to services to bringing services to patients", and suggested that professional registration and the development of practitioners in emergency care would support many of the paramedics who were keen to further expand their roles, suggesting that such roles would have wide support from the trade unions (Ambulance Services Association, 1999).

The clinical ramifications of these proposed changes were substantial, both operationally and professionally, since it was the paramedics upon whom a range of increasing responsibilities would fall. This role evolution was led not only by the phenomenon of rising patient demand but also by other important changes in the wider NHS, such as reconfigurations within primary care, including amendments to the contractual obligations of GPs in delivering care out of hours. In broad statistical terms, such changes have increased 999 call volumes from approximately one million in 1966 to nearly six million today with the largest increase of 3.2 million, in the order of 100%, occurring between 1996 and 2006.

The *Reforming Emergency Care* document (Department of Health, 2001) further developed the already established NHS Plan (Department of Health, 2000), setting the now familiar targets, including the recommendation of a 75%

ambulance response time for Category A (or life-threatening conditions) calls within eight minutes, although there remains scant scientific evidence for this apparently arbitrary time frame.

Development of emergency care practitioners roles

The right skill, right time, right place (Department of Health, 2004) document first outlined the role of the emergency care practitioner (ECP). This paper proposed the core competencies for the ECP role, although not a specific curriculum, as with other AHP advanced practice roles. Although initially viewed as helpful, many of the higher educational institutes involved in the pilot sites developed widely varying academic programmes, ranging from Level 2 to Masters level. This not only created confusion amongst the academic community but also subsequently on the clinical frontline. Patients could potentially receive varying standards of care, dependent on the practitioner's level of study and higher education institute. Clearly students studying at level 2 would have less depth of knowledge in a subject area than a student studying at Masters level. This issue of academic status was addressed at a later date, but often meant that further education and supervision were required for students who initially studied at a lower academic level.

The ECP role also had a profound influence on the developing profession of the paramedic. The ECP was, in reality, a parallel development championed by the now defunct Modernisation Agency which adopted the practitioner in emergency care concept and rebranded it as the ECP role. Similar in status to the practitioner in emergency care, the ECP thus dominated. The role of the ECP was aimed at meeting the demand for out-of-hours care provision, a service gap created by changes to the GP contract. A new approach to the academic preparation required for these paramedics, namely an educational as opposed to training approach, was challenging for many of these clinicians. Most paramedics, having undertaken the traditional IHCD programmes, despite having many years of clinical expertise, were yet to experience the adult-based learning of an academic education. Many paramedics undertaking the ECP programmes required additional study skills, effectively having to "learn how to learn"; most rose admirably to this challenge, embracing this new-found knowledge and learning, much to their credit.

Inexplicably, a contradictory and inconsistent decision was then made resulting in ECPs being promoted as the "new generic healthcare workers", which clearly they were not. With funding now largely ceased, the ECP consultation exercise was not universally well received, with objections from a number of high profile organisations including the JRCALC, the Higher Education Ambulance Development Group, the College of Paramedics, and others including the ambulance employers who had made individual and collective representation. In these circumstances the most charitable view of the ECP initiative would seem to indicate that it is an unnecessary, costly, confusing and wasteful duplication of effort to the initially proposed concept of a paramedic practitioner.

In 2003 the publication of *Ten key roles for Allied Health Professionals* aimed at clarifying the AHP role and what it should aim towards. It outlined that all AHPs should be able to act as the first point of contact for patient care having the skills of diagnosis, ordering diagnostic tests, prescribing, discharge, referral, teaching and health promotion (Department of Health, 2003)

The report by Hugo Minney (Department of Health, 2007) identified some of the key roles that ECPs (both nurses and paramedics) were undertaking. These roles included:

- *Out-of-hours services.* These services are employed as a mobile response to attend patients at home for primary care issues. Examples included managing primary care patients during the evening and weekends and responding to patients with potentially deteriorating long-term conditions such as cardiac and respiratory diseases and undertaking some home visits for GP services.
- *Ambulance service.* Many paramedic ECPs work from rapid or fast response vehicles to respond to, and manage "Category C" calls or calls to the ambulance service that are not deemed life-threatening and requiring an immediate response. ECPs were able to provide a safe, appropriate and effective treatment to a range of usually self-limiting illnesses and monitor conditions that do not require further treatment or transfer to hospital. Although there are limited data on the safety outcomes (Snooks et al, 2004; Mason et al, 2007) there does appear to be some financial benefit from the ECP model (Gray and Walker, 2008). However, since these ECPs worked as paramedics, they were able to utilise their professional expertise to identify and manage any patients who had been inaccurately categorised or who had deteriorated and required more urgent treatment.
- *Primary and community care.* During their academic programme, ECPs undertook clinical placements in GP surgeries and were often quickly able to manage "walk-ins" or patients requesting urgent same-day care. ECPs also managed home visits in-hours, in place of, but supervised by the GP, which allowed GPs more time to manage patients with more complex or serious conditions. Some GP practices were reluctant to part company with their ECP student, with some being offered posts on completion of their studies, testament to their usefulness and expertise. ECPs also worked in conjunction with other community care providers, such as district nurses, to provide complementary care, following referral from the ambulance service (Venstone and Wade, 2005).
- *Emergency departments, walk-in clinics and urgent care centres.* Typically ECPs also had clinical placements in all these facilities (or

similar) and whilst there is little evidence regarding the subsequent impact on clinical care, the role undoubtedly afforded ECPs with ample clinical experience of patients presenting with a range of conditions that may have otherwise requested an ambulance, and that they could apply in their future clinical practice.

Taking healthcare to the patient (Department of Health, 2005), also referred to as the Bradley Report, made a virtue out of necessity in recommending that the ambulance service take on the responsibilities of a mobile healthcare provider, with the broad objective of reducing the number of patient transports to hospital by approximately 25%, or roughly one million journeys per annum. Ambulance services and their staff have embraced this challenge, which has also been endorsed by the College of Paramedics.

Whilst professional development of paramedics was welcomed, there will always be debate with regard to the skills and competencies that paramedics require, and rightly so, since debate and discussion are essential for the professional development of the paramedic role. The JRCALC clinical guidelines provide an advisory evidence-based framework for practice. These guidelines outline clinical paramedic practice and include recommendations for administration of a range of therapeutic agents (JRCALC, 2006; 2009). As with most developing professions, opinions regarding best practice vary over time; therapeutic regimes and emergency and urgent care guidelines are amended on a regular basis as a result of clinical expertise and research evidence. For example the paramedic role in the treatment and management of a suspected acute myocardial infarction is a classic example of changes to paramedic practice based on evidence that directly impacts patient care. The safe administration of thrombolytic therapy in the urgent care setting has been proven beneficial, reducing both morbidity and mortality (JRCALC, 2004; Khan et al, 2009), and this has been superseded in some areas by percutaneous coronary interventions or angioplasty, which alleviate symptoms and decrease morbidity and mortality (Chittari et al, 2005; Johnston et al, 2006).

Paramedic education

In common with all other AHPs administered by the Health Professions Council, educational standards have been set in the *Standards of Education and Training* (Health Professions Council, 2009). This document guides university curricula and assessment standards and supports the validation process. Similarly the Health Professions Council's *Standards of Proficiency* (2007–9) with generic and profession-specific standards, states that all paramedics should undertake full patient assessment, possess clinical reasoning skills and refer patients appropriately. In addition the Quality

Assurance Agency (2004) *Subject Benchmark Statements*, developed at the request of the Department of Health, apply a number of benchmark statements to all academic healthcare programmes (see *Table 1:1*). The Health Professions Council clearly identified that paramedics should have the competency set to meet patient demand, and specifically to enhance patient assessment and clinical decision-making – all required to support graduate paramedics and advanced roles, such as ECPs. This marked a significant shift from the existing didactic training approach of the IHCD, which falls far short of preparing paramedics for advanced practice.

The Quality Assurance Agency set out clear criteria for any new occupations wishing to seek registration. They included guidance on the aspect of the role that should, amongst others issues, encompass a defined body of knowledge, carry out evidence-based practice, be part of an established professional body and should have a commitment to continuing professional development.

The Healthcare Quality Improvement Partnership was established in 2008 with an aim of promoting quality in healthcare and specifically to increase the impact of clinical audit on healthcare quality in England and Wales. Led by a consortium of the Academy of Royal Colleges, the Royal College of Nursing and National Voices (formerly the Long-Term Conditions Alliance), the Healthcare Quality Improvement Partnership works in with healthcare stakeholders to improve quality in healthcare, promote value for money and enable a culture of quality improvement.

One of the Healthcare Quality Improvement Partnership's associated groups is the National Ambulance Clinical Audit Steering Group. This Steering Group aims to support the strategic development and coordination of clinical audit and quality improvement in the ambulance services, thereby encouraging a coherent, consistent framework for clinical audit. The Steering Group is also aiming to increase the capacity, skills and techniques for clinical quality improvement in the ambulance services.

The establishment of continuing professional development (CPD) remains a relatively new concept for paramedics. CPD is now a requirement of Health Professions Council registered paramedics, and is perhaps more important in the development of advanced practice, such as is carried out by ECPs. It has long been suggested that ECPs (who should now correctly be referred to as paramedic practitioners) should have a separate registerable qualification. Some critics argue that this would lead to unnecessary bureaucracy and is redundant as paramedics (and nurses), from whom the vast majority of these advanced practitioners are drawn, are already subject to registration. However it is a well-established fact that as any professional group matures and evolves to meet new challenges, there is a need to generate new professional groups. Since the paramedic profession does have a unique skill set, this argument will be debated for some time to come.

Table 1.1. Quality Assurance Agency Paramedic Benchmark Statements (QAA, 2004)

A: The paramedic as a registered health care practitioner: Expectations held by the profession, employers and the public

A1: Professional identity autonomy and accountability of the paramedic

A2: Professional relationships relating to paramedic practice

A3: Personal and professional skills

A4: Profession and employer context for the practice of paramedics

B: Paramedic skills and their application to practice

B1: Patient assessment

B2: Application of paramedic practice
- formulation of plans and strategies for meeting health and social care needs

B3: Evaluation of paramedic practice

C: Paramedic science: Subject knowledge, understanding and associated skills

C1: Scientific basis of paramedic practice
- biological, behavioural and clinical sciences

C2: Context of service delivery and professional practice
- service/organisation issues
- social and political
- ethical and moral dimensions

Specific knowledge, understanding and associated skills that underpin the education and training of paramedic scientists

Paramedic practice

Natural and life sciences

Social, health and behavioural sciences

Ethics, laws and humanities

Management of self and other's reflective practice

Associated skills
- communication and interpersonal skills
- information gathering
- care delivery
- problem solving, data collection and interpretation
- information technology
- numeracy

Academic requirements for paramedic practice

As highlighted earlier, there has been a growing trend towards academic university-based programmes for paramedics, such as undergraduate and foundation degrees, offered on a full and part-time basis, delivered by a number of higher education institutes in the UK. There are currently a number of first and second level degree awards available to paramedics, including Bachelor (Honours) degrees in paramedic science and pre-hospital care, with a small but growing number of paramedics undertaking Masters degrees.

To support the advancing paramedic practice and the developing academic reconfiguration required for such roles, the College of Paramedics published its *Curriculum Guidance and Competence Framework* (2008) (see *Figure 1:1*). This revised framework followed wide stakeholder input. It also outlines a scope of practice and career framework for specialist, advanced and consultant paramedics – roles that are becoming increasingly commonplace within ambulance trusts. The identified competencies require further clarification and discussion and, whilst theoretically are relatively easy to identify, their application and assessment is more challenging and will continue to be reviewed.

One recent example of the development of the paramedic role is that of the critical care paramedic. The core academic curriculum for the critical care paramedic is drawn from concepts of nursing knowledge, theories, trauma and surgical care, and anaesthetics, much of which has been adapted to form the basis of the critical care paramedic programmes. Similar to some of the nurse practitioner development, the critical care paramedic role originated from the Department of Health's New Ways of Working programmes that were initially developed for critical care practitioners, which aimed to develop hospital nurses working in critical care and intensive care units. One of the New Ways of Working pilot projects, the critical care paramedic academic programme at the University of Hertfordshire, initially offered an opportunity to extrapolate and explore some of the critical care issues in the pre-hospital setting, specifically in relation to inter-hospital transfers, which often negatively impacted on the in-hospital critical care staff who were frequently required to accompany critically ill patients for such transfers. This was also in line with the developments in pre-hospital, immediate and traumatic care.

The critical care paramedic programmes initially offered air ambulance paramedics the opportunity to develop and advance their existing knowledge, skills and attributes in order to increase the capacity of care provision whilst continuing to improve the quality of care in this specialised setting. This particular area of paramedic practice will undoubtedly become increasingly popular, developing the critical care aspect of the paramedic role along with the primary care developments seen in the ECP role.

Paramedic practice today

Other developments in the paramedic role have been in that of management. In the earlier days of practice, the operational management of paramedics was by a medical director who controlled and oversaw all clinical practice, with paramedics calling into a local hospital and receiving orders for every individual procedure or drug that was required. Clearly this was both cumbersome and time-consuming. As physicians began to build trust in paramedics during their experience of working with them, confidence levels rose. Increasingly day-to-day operations moved from direct and immediate medical control to pre-written

(9)	Clinical Director of Service	Senior staff with ultimate accountability, management and co-ordination of out-of-hospital unscheduled, pre-hospital care
(8)	Consultant Practitioners	These practitioners have expertise in practice, involvement in education, research and strategic and professional leadership with allied health professions' criteria for consultant roles
(7)	Advanced Practitioners	Experienced paramedics with advanced clinical or educational knowledge following postgraduate study
(6)	Senior Practitioners/Specialist Practitioners	Paramedics with a higher degree of autonomy who have specialised in a specific area of clinical or educational practice following further study at level 6 in a relevant science degree
(5)	Practitioners	Paramedics at the beginning of their professional career. They will be able to examine and assess patient's acute and chronic condition, record a full history, treat to a specific level and appropriately refer within their scope of practice following education at level 5 (Diploma)
(4)	Assistant Practitioners/Associate Practitioners	The development of support roles to work alongside paramedics has been implemented nationally. These people will provide support to and be guided by qualified ambulance practitioners. They may occasionally be required to provide immediate resuscitative measures in case of acute, immediately life-threatening conditions until more qualified help arrives.
(3)	Senior Healthcare Assistants/ Technicians	
(2)	Support Workers	
(1)	Initial Entry Level Jobs	

Figure 1.1. College of Paramedics' career framework.

protocols or "standing orders" with the paramedic typically only calling in for direction after the options in the standing orders had been exhausted.

Paramedics are now frequently seen in a range of middle and senior management roles, providing daily support for front-line staff of all levels, managing clinical workloads and, increasingly, providing clinical leadership at an executive board level. A number of academic management and leadership programmes have developed to support paramedics in such roles. As paramedics became increasingly professionalised, working in a range of clinical settings and continuing to evolve and develop, the lack of an appropriate peer-reviewed journal was becoming increasingly obvious. The recently launched *Journal of Paramedic Practice* is testament to the developing professional status of the paramedic. The journal works closely with the College of Paramedics and others, with the objective of encouraging and supporting paramedics in their clinical, professional and academic development. Other future developments include the College of Paramedics gaining Royal status, with the ability to suggest and support legislation, lobby for policy change, set exams, deal with complaints and so on, as with other health professional bodies. The JRCALC guidelines will continue to be reviewed and updated, striving to develop and support clinical and autonomous practice.

There is a growing trend for professionalisation of paramedic practice, with their increasing academic preparation and their collaborative working with other HCPs in a range of clinical settings. Such interdisciplinary working and shared practice, largely unexplored phenomena in paramedic practice, will help to remove some of the barriers that have tended to ring-fence the ambulance service as a Cinderella service.

Specialist registration

The continued expansion of practice could most usefully be recognised through the provision of a "specialist's register", similar to the nursing and medical profession and/or as an annotation to primary registration. The professional bodies' prime directive of ensuring public protection through clarifying which practitioners have undergone accredited training and education in a particular clinical area, could be effectively recognised without the need for separate or additional registration, although such suggestions are still being discussed. The College of Paramedics is discussing setting up a voluntary annotated register for extended/advanced scope of practice, with the support of the Health Professions Council, who could take over this responsibility at some point in the future. This register will list those practising to benchmark standards laid out in the various specialist areas and will greatly assist in supporting the implementation of the paramedic career framework. Paramedics operating in these new roles could usefully set the benchmarks and ensure that other safeguards are established.

Specialist roles

Paramedics now work in a range of areas, the vast majority for NHS ambulance services, in a number of different roles such as general frontline care and more specialised roles including Hazardous Material Teams, Urban Search and Rescue Teams or Hazardous Area Response Teams. Whilst many paramedics have undertaken a managerial role, other paramedics have been employed in education and teaching roles, becoming university lecturers on the range of paramedic degree programmes. Less commonly they have become lecturer-practitioners, undertaking a joint role with the local NHS ambulance trust and higher educational institute thereby providing credible and much needed support for students in clinical placement.

There is also an increasing trend for the role of consultant paramedic, as highlighted in the College of Paramedics' *Curriculum Guidance and Competence Framework* (2008). The first UK consultant paramedic was appointed in South East Coast Ambulance Service NHS Trust and performs the role of clinical director, and is co-author of the first chapter of this book. The first professor of paramedics was recently appointed at Coventry University and this, in addition to similar roles in the UK and Australia, are vital in developing the much-needed research base for paramedic practice.

As highlighted earlier, a number of paramedics work with the air ambulance service, which, although funded through private, charitable donations, is clinically governed and employed by local NHS ambulance trusts. A number work as paramedic practitioners in an out-of-hours role, attached to a primary care trust or GP surgery, delivering and complementing some of the care previously undertaken by GPs. Some paramedics work with private ambulance services, the prison service, and event organisation companies; some support military operations, including assistance with medical evacuation; some provide emergency care in mining and remote industrial settings and oil rigs; and others work with the police.

Paramedic prescribing

One of the key issues to support future practice will be paramedic prescribing. Unlike nurses and other AHPs, currently paramedics are unable to access any of the non-medical prescribing educational programmes, such as supplementary and independent prescribing (as described in *Chapter 2*). However, paramedics are able to administer medications for a range of clinical conditions, as outlined in the JRCALC Guidelines. This has resulted in the administration by paramedics of opiate analgesia and a range of cardiac, respiratory and gastrointestinal drugs. Historically IHCD technician and paramedic training programmes have provided very little in the way of an underpinning framework of pharmacological principles and concepts in preparation for the administration of these drugs. Whilst these are a necessity for the management of the urgent, and often life-limiting conditions which present to paramedics on a daily basis, there does appear to be a dichotomy between the administration of drugs by paramedics and other AHPs. There are plans in the future to extend non-medical prescribing to paramedics, although no specific date is planned. Release from practice for training will inevitably be an issue and some higher educational institutes have adapted a number of their existing programmes to incorporate online and/or blended learning that will address some of the issues. However a positive aspect will be the shared learning that these generic AHP programmes will offer.

Higher educational institute programmes for paramedic practitioner training, such as the ECP and critical care paramedic, do have a pharmacology content. This particular aspect of education, with which some paramedic students often struggle, is welcomed, providing much-needed underpinning theory. Such was the didactic nature of the traditional training of paramedics that often there was little time and no explicit need for such knowledge, to the detriment of paramedics and their patients.

The future of pre-hospital care

With the increasing variety and complexity of paramedic roles, the NHS Career Framework considers such AHPs to be working beyond career framework level 5 (the initial registration level) as specialist/senior or advanced practitioners (see *Table 1.2*).

As such, many NHS employers have adopted a number of terms to describe these roles, such as, advanced paramedic practitioners, community paramedics, community paramedic officers (Department of Health, 2003), paramedic practitioners, senior practitioners and, most unhelpfully of all, ECPs. This is unhelpful because of the confusion surrounding the original practitioner in emergency care role and the wide range of similar nursing roles. In such cases it is usually the relevant professional body that would be the logical reference point and the College of Paramedics has provided guidance on this matter.

All professions need to evolve and, given the nature of the current ambulance service particularly in the pre-hospital setting, a number of differing developments across the UK ensure that patient need is met. Fundamentally with further education, paramedics have developed into practitioners who have extended their scope of practice beyond the minimum standards of proficiency for registration. Generally these developments have been in primary care, aimed at increasing the paramedic's ability to deal effectively with patients in the community to reduce the number of inappropriate hospital admissions and, in some cases, to support early hospital discharge. However these developments have, as described, also occurred in neonatal and critical care.

Any sound initiative that enhances the scope of paramedic practice to

Table 1.2. Applied qualifications framework for paramedics			
Grade of paramedic	*Educational award*	*Clinical context*	*Academic level*
Consultant paramedic	Doctorate	Clinical and organisational leaders Experts in practice	8
Advanced paramedic	Masters Degree Postgraduate Diploma Postgraduate Certificate	Extended scope of practice Detailed understanding of complex body of knowledge Apply clinical judgement and advanced clinical experience in decision-making	7
Specialist paramedic	Bachelor Degree Graduate Diploma Graduate Certificate	Proficient, coordinated and confident Able to examine and assess patients	6
Paramedic	Foundation Degree Diploma of Higher Education Diploma of Further Education Higher National Diploma Level 5 BTEC Higher National Diploma	Primary registration with Health Professions Council Clinically safe to work alone	5
Adapted from College of Paramedics (2008b)			

meet changing patient need should be welcomed, with the proviso that this work should only be countenanced when there are appropriate safeguards and mechanisms in place to ensure that additional responsibilities can be discharged safely and effectively. The following points underpin the management, development and implementation of the career framework and regulation for the paramedic profession:

• Development of scope of practice is a natural progression as a professional and is clearly articulated via the continuing professional development process.

- The profession nurtures a sound evidence base for practice and it must develop experts within the field.
- A body of knowledge for extensions to paramedic practice should be constructed and owned within the profession.
- The development of extended scope of practice for paramedics will serve both patients and the health economy within the range of demands placed on ambulance services.
- The creation and separate regulation of "new" professions that would have a better, more natural fit as an extended scope of practice for existing professions should be discouraged.
- Any extension of clinical practice occurs in partnership with the relevant medical and other specialists to ensure the widest possible level of support to foster an environment where interprofessional teamwork, mentorship and coaching can thrive.
- A specialist annotation to the primary register is the most effective means of standardising, regulating and identifying paramedics with an extended scope of practice.

The term specialist paramedic, as supported by the NHS Career Framework, provides a useful reference point to aid standardisation, as having similar role titles across the country enhances collaboration, patient awareness, and interprofessional liaison. The term should be accompanied by identification of specific specialist areas as they are developed, e.g. specialist paramedic (primary care). This job title structure should be used to replace the wide variety of titles for specialist paramedics currently used across ambulance trusts.

Conclusion

It is clear that as a profession develops it is natural for specialist areas to emerge and for individuals to become expert in areas of professional knowledge in response to the demands and requirements of healthcare provision. Inevitably this growth and expansion of role will to some extent encroach upon other professionals' territory. With luck this can be successfully navigated, but there is always a risk that other professionals will react in a negative way and it is not always possible to rely upon a positive reaction. In such times it is helpful to turn to "reference points" such as the paramedic career structure and to adopt a unified approach to designations and nomenclature to help resolve any lack of clarity that may be present.

References

Ambulance Service Association (1999) *The future of the Ambulance Service in the UK 2000–2010*. London: Ambulance Services Association

Bissell R, Seaman KG, Bass R, Racht CG, Welgate A, F. Doctor M, Moriarity S, Eslinger D, Doherty R (1999) Change the scope of practice of paramedics? *Prehospital Emergency Care* **3**(2): 140–9

Chamberlain D (2000) *The future role and education of paramedic ambulance service personnel (emerging concepts)*. London: JRCALC/ Ambulance Services Association.

Chittari MSVM, Ahmad I, Chambers B, Knight F, Scriven A, Pitcher D (2005) Retrospective observational case-control study comparing prehospital thrombolytic therapy for ST-elevation myocardial infarction with in-hospital thrombolytic therapy for patient from same area. *Emergency Medicine Journal* **22**(8): 582–5

College of Paramedics (2008) *Curriculum Guidance and Competence Framework*. London: College of Paramedics

Department of Health (1946) *National Health Service Act*. London: HMSO

Department of Health (1997) *Developing Emergency Services in the Community – Final Report*. London: HMSO.

Department of Health (2000) *The NHS Plan. A plan for investment. A plan for reform*. London: HMSO

Department of Health (2001) *Reforming emergency care in England – First steps to a new approach*. London: HMSO

Department of Health (2003) *Allied health professions with a specialist interest*. London: HMSO

Department of Health (2004) *Right skill, right time, right place*. London: HMSO

Department of Health (2005) *Taking healthcare to the patient – Transforming NHS ambulance services*. London: HMSO.

Department of Health (2007) *Measuring the benefits of the emergency care practitioner*. London: HMSO.

Dunne RB, Compton S, Welch RD, Zalenski RJ, Bock BF (2003) Prehospital onsite triaging. *Prehospital Emergency Care* **7**(2): 85–8.

Geddes JS (1986) Twenty years of pre-hospital coronary care. *British Heart Journal* **56**(6): 491–5

Gray JT, Walker A (2008) Avoiding admissions from the ambulance service: A review of elderly patients with falls and patients with breathing difficulties seen by emergency care practitioners in South Yorkshire. *Emergency Medical Journal* **25**(3): 168–71

Health Professions Council (2007-9) *Standards of proficiency*. London: HPC.

Health Professions Council (2009) *Standards of education and training*. London: HPC.

Johnston S, Brightwell R, Ziman M (2006) Paramedics and pre-hospital management of acute myocardial infarction: Diagnosis and reperfusion. *Emergency Medical Journal* 23(4): 331–4

JRCALC (2004) *Prehospital thrombolytic therapy JRCALC Position Statement: July 2004.* Warwick: JRCALC.

JRCALC (2006) *UK ambulance service clinical practice guidelines.* Warwick: JRCALC.

JRCALC (2009) *Clinical practice guideline updates post-2006 publication of the UK Ambulance Service Clinical Practice Guidelines (2006).* Warwick: JRCALC

JRCALC and the Ambulance Service Association (2000) *The future role and education of paramedic ambulance service personnel (emerging concepts).* Warwick: JRCALC

Khan SN, Murray P, McCormick L, Sharples LS, Salahshouri P, Scott J, Schofield PM (2009) Paramedic-led prehospital thrombolysis is safe and effective: The East Anglian experience. *Emergency Medicine Journal* 26(6): 452–5

Kilner T (2004) Desirable attributes of the ambulance technician, paramedic and clinical supervisor: Findings of a Delphi study. *Emergency Medicine Journal* 21(3): 374–8

Mason S, O'Keefe C, Coleman P, Edlin R, Nicholl J (2007) Effectiveness of emergency care practitioners working in the existing emergency service models of care. *Emergency Medicine Journal* 24(4): 239–43

Ministry of Health, Scottish Home and Health Department (1966) *Report by the working party on ambulance training and equipment: Part 1—training.* London: HMSO

Ministry of Health, Scottish Home and Health Department (1967) *Report by the working party on ambulance training and equipment: Part 2—equipment and vehicles.* London: HMSO

National Academy of Sciences (1966) *Accidental death and disability: The neglected disease of modern society.* Washington DC: National Research Council

Palazzo FF, Warner OJ, Harron M, Morrison WG (1998) Misuse of the London Ambulance Service: How much and why? *Journal of Accident and Emergency Medicine* 15(6): 368–70

Quality Assurance Agency (2004) *Benchmark statements: Healthcare programmes – paramedic science.* Gloucester: QAA

Schmidt T, Atcheson R, Federiuk C, Clay Mann N, Pinney T, Fuller D, Colbry K (2000) Evaluation of protocols allowing emergency medical technicians to determine the need for treatment and transport. *Academic*

Emergency Medicine **7**(6): 663–9

Snooks H, Kearsley N, Dale J, Halter M, Redhead J, Cheung WY (2004) Towards primary care for non-serious 999 callers: Results of a controlled study of "treat and refer" protocols for ambulance crews. *Quality and Safety in Health Care* **13**(6): 435–43

Venstone G, Wade E (2005) *Luton and Dunstable Hospital Accident and Emergency study* (unpublished report)

CHAPTER 2

Nursing practice

History of the nursing profession

The history of nursing dates back to a time when "medical" care was provided in religious temples and churches and often by women. This is perhaps the origin of the term "sister" for a senior, female nurse. These women often had little, if any, training, relying on folklore and the use of herbs and plants to assist with various ailments. Women then moved to delivering care within the home – the first district or community nurses – gaining valuable experience in managing a vast range of disease and infection, as well as assisting women in childbirth.

Florence Nightingale and Mary Seacole

Historically the most well-known nursing pioneer was Florence Nightingale (1820–1910), who is considered one of the founders of nursing theory. In the late 19th century, the insanitary conditions in all hospitals were an enormous health hazard. Nightingale correctly concluded, through early statistical research, that external factors were pivotal to mortality and morbidity rates. This was revolutionary at the time since nurses were employed simply to undertake tasks, certainly not to think, research and publish their findings. Although now highly regarded and respected, during her nursing career Nightingale's research was largely ignored by the Government of the day.

Nightingale is perhaps best known for her work during the Crimean War in the 1850s where she and several colleagues travelled to the war zone and were appalled at the conditions in which the wounded were being cared for. Overwhelming infections, such as typhus, cholera and dysentery, were contaminating the soldiers wounds and accounting for almost 20% of all deaths.

Nightingale's radical reformation of these field hospitals, using simple yet effective measures to improve the sanitary conditions, dramatically reduced mortality and morbidity.

Following the war in 1856, Nightingale returned to England a national heroine. Greatly moved by the lack of basic sanitation and nursing care of the Crimean soldiers, she began a campaign to improve the quality of nursing in all military and civilian hospitals. In 1860 a nursing school bearing her name was set up at St Thomas' Hospital, London in the UK. Although less popular in her later years, Nightingale will remain forever fixed in the public memory as a heroine of the Crimean War and, to many, the founder of the nursing profession through her research and her ardent campaigning for a woman's right to a nursing career which was frowned upon in the paternalistic society of the day (Nightingale, 1969).

Another historically important nursing figure was Mary Seacole (1805– 1881). This Jamaican-born British nurse was, like Florence Nightingale, also known for her involvement in the Crimean War. On hearing of the poor nursing care in the Crimean field hospitals, Seacole was convinced her knowledge of tropical medicine could be beneficial and she volunteered as a nurse. Seacole treated wounded soldiers from both sides of the conflict, often while under fire. Nightingale's work over-shadowed Seacole's contribution and the latter was somewhat forgotten until, more recently, when she has been remembered for her nursing skills and bravery.

The National Health Service

The NHS was set up following the National Health Service Act 1946 (Department of Health, 1946) to provide healthcare to anyone normally resident in the United Kingdom, the majority of services being free at the point of use. Lauded, idealistically perhaps, as the "envy of the world" the NHS was based on the long-held belief that good healthcare should be available to all, regardless of wealth. When launched, the then Health Minister, Aneurin Bevan, stated that the NHS should have three core principles:

1. To meet the needs of everyone.
2. To be free at the point of delivery.
3. To be based on clinical need, not ability to pay.

The role of nurses in healthcare delivery precedes the NHS of course with many nurses and "midwives" administering care in the community for centuries prior to its inception. Unregulated and uneducated though these nurses were, they formed the basis of some of today's nursing practice. Nursing as a profession has developed rapidly over the past 40 years, with changes to nurse education from hospital-based training to university-based academic programmes offering diplomas, degrees and doctorates.

Nursing regulation and registration

The nursing profession in the UK is overseen nationally by the Chief Nursing Officer, employed by the Department of Health, to provide guidance to the Government on matters relating to nursing practice. Nursing's professional body is the Royal College of Nursing (RCN), which represents qualified and student nurses and aims to promote excellence in nursing through practice and shaping health policies. The RCN also provides an educational role, lobbies Government on policy, and raises the profile of nursing in the UK.

The Nursing and Midwifery Council (NMC) was established in 2002 as nursing's statutory body, under the Nursing and Midwifery Order (Office of Public Sector Information, 2001a). The NMC replaced the English National Board for Nursing, Midwifery and Health Visiting (ENB) as the UK regulator for nursing and midwifery. The NMC's aim is to protect the public by ensuring that nurses and midwives provide high standards of care, and it maintains a register of qualified nurses, midwives and health visitors in the UK. It sets standards for education, practice and conduct, provides advice for nurses, midwives and health visitors and considers allegations of misconduct or unfitness to practise due to ill health. In 2008 the NMC (2008a) published *The Code – Standards of conduct, performance and ethics for nurses and midwives*.

The mid-19th to early 20th century witnessed the state registration of the medical profession with debate that a similar system was required for nurses. In the 1880s Ethel Bedford-Fenwick, Matron at St Bartholomew's Hospital, felt strongly that nursing should be more closely aligned to the medical profession, establishing what is currently the International Council of Nurses (ICN) and the *British Journal of Nursing*. Bedford-Fenwick significantly extended the nurse's role and campaigned for the state registration of nurses. *Table 2.1* outlines many of the key historical events of the 20th and 21st century. Whilst this list in not exhaustive, it does provide a brief snapshot of some of the key events that have guided nursing development over the years.

As nursing has evolved, a growing number of specialist nursing roles have developed, some to meet the demand of patient care and some to meet the gap in demand created by changes to the roles of other healthcare providers. One specific, and much debated, example of the development in the role of nurses is NHS Direct. NHS Direct was introduced in 1997 as a 24-hour nurse-led telephone helpline service aimed at providing the public with accessible information and advice regarding health and illness, with an emphasis on self-care. NHS Direct currently receives approximately 5 million calls annually over 36 sites (Department of Health, 2009a). Although criticised by some for the lack of positive impact on reducing pressure on other urgent care services, such as the ambulance service, NHS Direct does represent the formal recognition of some collaborative working between nurses and paramedics, with many NHS Direct centres situated within ambulance trusts (Mayor, 2000; Munro et al, 2000; Heyworth, 2001; Peacock et al, 2005).

Many of these specialist nursing roles are associated with advanced practice – nurses pushing the boundaries of practice and undertaking skills and competencies previously undertaken by doctors. *Table 2.2* outlines some examples of the development of nursing roles and titles. Many of these nurses work within the urgent or pre-hospital care setting, such as walk-in centres,

Table 2.1. Key health events of the 20th century	
Date	Event
1910–20	Forerunner of the current RCN established (1916) Nurses Registration Act (1919)
1920–30	First nurse tutor role and state nurse examinations
1930–40	Formal recognition of the State Enrolled Nurse
1940–50	Formation of the NHS (1946)
1950–60	Mental Health Act Introduction of tranquilising agents in mental health care
1960–70	Availability and use of sterile dressing, syringes and the sterilisation of medical equipment First professor of nursing appointed at Manchester University RCN becomes a trade union University of Edinburgh provides the first nursing degree
1970–80	Briggs Committee Report (1972) recommends unified council, rather than the existing four separate country boards, to regulate education Nurses, Midwives and Health Visitors Act (1979)
1980–90	UKCC becomes nursing's new professional body (1983) to oversee educational quality assurance and maintain training records
1990–99	NHS Direct launched (1997) (Department of Health, 1997b)
2000	Introduction of Project 2000 Enrolled nurse training ceases (with later conversion courses developed for SENs) University-based nursing programmes start NHS Plan (Department of Health, 2000) sets out a number of healthcare reforms National Institute for Clinical Excellence (NICE) is set up
2004	Agenda for Change published (Department of Health, 2004a; c)
2005	Bradley Report published (Department of Health, 2005)
2006	Knowledge and Skills Framework (KSF) published, applicable to all healthcare roles Ambulance trusts merge
2008	Darzi Review published (Department of Health, 2008)

minor injury units and urgent care centres. The aim of these facilities is to reduce the number of patients attending emergency departments, specifically those with primary care health issues, such as minor self-limiting illnesses and injuries and some health prevention issues. Theoretically this reduces the pressure on emergency departments so that they can concentrate on managing patients who require the services of a full emergency department facility, such as patients with major trauma or life-threatening or serious illness. These facilities may be co-located within or near the emergency department or at a separate geographical site. Those located within or near the emergency department have triaged patients referred to them via the usual screening mechanism, often a triage desk (or nurse). This is effective in screening patients whose health needs can best be met by nurse practitioners or those in a similar advanced role. With the essential additional competence in non-medical prescribing, many patients avoid emergency departments entirely.

Many emergency care practitioner (ECP) students anecdotally found their placements in these nurse-led environments extremely useful for their learning and development. This was largely due to the similarity in the role of the nurse practitioner and ECP, specifically in terms of patient management, as many of the treatment and assessment skills are easily transferred to the pre-hospital setting. In addition the development of these relationships facilitated future networking once the ECP students had graduated – knowledge of these personnel and the available resources and expertise ensured that patients the ECPs were unable to manage in the pre-hospital setting could be referred directly into an emergency department.

A clinical example would be that of the management of a laceration. The vast majority of lacerations can be successfully closed with either skin closure dressings (such as Steri-strips) or a skin tissue adhesive (such as Histoacryl). Since these products are small and portable and can stored at ambient temperatures, lacerations can be managed effectively in the pre-hospital setting. However deeper lacerations, potentially with a retained foreign body or with tendon or ligament damage, require further exploration and traditional suturing. This is usually outside the clinical practice of an ECP or paramedic practitioner and such patients need to attend an emergency department. Such referrals can be directed straight to an appropriate healthcare practitioner within the emergency department (often a nurse practitioner) since the patient's history, examination and key treatments have often already been completed. This is a good example of where the two professions overlap and contribute to patient care. *Table 2.2* also outlines examples of nursing roles that are related to the urgent/pre-hospital setting.

Nurse education

The training of nurses has undergone many changes over the past 50 years. Dame Catherine Hall, RCN General Secretary 1957–1982, lobbied strongly for the recognition of the professional status of nursing and for improved standards of nursing care. In 1964, the RCN reported to the Platt Committee on education,

Table 2.2. Examples of nursing roles related to urgent/pre-hospital care

Role and title	Area of work	Clinical area	Training/education
Nurse practitioners: advanced clinical nurses, emergency nurse practitioners, first contact practitioners	Work in primary and urgent care: emergency departments, minor injury clinics, walk-in centres	Minor injury/illness: chest infections, influenza, coughs and colds, minor wounds, falls, sprains, minor uncomplicated digit fractures, etc.	BSc or Diploma in their clinical speciality
Specialist community public health nurses: district nurses, school nurses	Primary and community: often part of intermediate care teams, facilitate early discharge or admission prevention, particularly in patients with long-term conditions and older patients	Wound management, child health and wellbeing, health and social care of patients with long-term conditions and older patients, etc.	BSc with additional postgraduate course in their area of expertise
Clinical nurse specialists: working in specialist clinical areas	Work either in primary care, attached to a GP surgery or part of a primary care trust or in secondary care as part of a multidisciplinary hospital-based specialist team, often providing lay community clinics. Often support early discharge/admission avoidance programmes	Autonomously manage patients with long-term conditions such as respiratory, cardiac, dermatology, diabetic, rheumatology, trauma cardiovascular, palliative care, etc.	BSc or MSc in their subject area

Nurse consultants: can also be called consultant nurses	Can work in any clinical area similar to that of the clinical nurse specialist and have an additional remit of education and research	May work in emergency departments alongside medical colleagues in any of the specialities listed for clinical nurse specialists, the key difference being the research aspect to their role	MSc PhD
Lecturer practitioners: sometimes joint appointment between a trust and higher education institute	Based in a higher education institute and working collaboratively between the NHS and the higher education institute to support students in clinical practice	Provide teaching and mentorship for students in the clinical setting, whilst delivering academic sessions/tutorials within the higher education institute	Certificate/Diploma in teaching in Higher Education BSc/MSc May be working towards a PhD
Lecturers: senior and principal lecturers	Based in a higher education institute, they teach a range of subjects related to their clinical experience, and undertake research	Usually derived from the speciality in which they teach, e.g. emergency department nurses teaching on trauma and emergency nurse practitioner programmes	Certificate/Diploma in teaching in Higher Education Profession-related BSc/MSc

stating that nurses in training should have student nurse status and that schools of nursing should be separate from hospital. Although student status was not achieved for a number of years following Dame Hall's retirement, she helped to lay the foundations for nurse education for the following 30 years.

During the 1980s the two existing statutory bodies in nursing, the UKCC and the ENB, with the RCN, underwent a fundamental change in their approach to nurse training. Nurses were required to take responsibility for their professional development and they acquired competencies rather than learned them from explicitly defined content and structured nurse training. Education as opposed to training would be on a self-directed basis, and competencies would be acquired through applied knowledge, skills and attributes linked to a nursing model that focused on health rather than illness (Bradshaw, 1997). The curriculum content was to be broad, including social and political health-related factors, with practical skills being acquired under an identified "mentor" in a supernumerary approach. This of course is the recognisable path that paramedics are beginning to undertake.

Student examination and assessment was to be the responsibility of the individual educational institutions, no longer a central body as before. The UKCC, as the then registrant organisation, would expect those seeking registration to demonstrate their competencies in order to practise. What was less clear was how the competencies would be measured. The intended outcome of this new training would be a "knowledgeable doer". Despite some noted divisions defining the role of the nurse and the regulatory certification and accountability required for professional advancement, the new training structure was formalised as Project 2000 with the Common Foundation Programme (CFP) and the branch programmes leading to registration. Competency was to be assessed through learning outcomes with continuous assessment being recommended for theoretical and practical aspects of the course. As such, nurse education was based on nurses defining and assessing their own standards of competency. This is challenging when those competencies are neither defined nor tested, thereby questioning the underpinning preparation that was aimed for in the paradigm shift from training to education (Bradshaw, 1998; Bradshaw and Merriman, 2008).

Students successfully qualifying from these programmes became State Registered Nurses (SRNs) – later changed to Registered General Nurses (RGNs) – and were registered with the UKCC, now the NMC. The SEN role was phased out, with many SENs converting to RGNs via various academic conversion programmes. "Basic" nursing skills are now performed by an unqualified or vocationally trained healthcare assistant (HCA) or assistant practitioner (AP), who may lack exposure to some core clinical skills.

Today, strategic health authorities have contracts with local NHS trusts and hospitals and negotiate with higher education institutes to deliver academic programmes for a contracted number of students, including paramedics, physiotherapists and occupational therapists amongst others. The delivery of nurse education is entirely within higher education institutes, which generally provide training and education in all branches of nursing (adult, child, mental health and learning disability) with programmes having a 50/50 split between theory and practice. The latter is undertaken in a range of clinical settings. The core curriculum for nurses now comprises a year's programme where nursing students are taught the generic, core knowledge and theory underpinning all branches of nursing, such as anatomy and physiology, applied pathophysiology, communication, social policy, and pharmacology. The second and third years focus on the knowledge, theory and practice required for the branch of choice. Whilst midwifery and health visiting are regarded as separate professions, they are still within the nursing family, the latter requiring a basic nurse education as a foundation.

All courses are validated by the NMC (2004) and have to conform to the relevant standards outlined by the Quality Assurance Agency's Standards and Benchmark Statements (2008).

Post-registration education and changes to salary structures

Following qualification, the NMC requires nurses to undertake at least 35 hours of education every three years in order to remain up to date as part of the Post-Registration Education and Practice (PREP) requirements (NMC, 2008b). Nurses also frequently undertake a range of additional programmes of study to develop further their skills and/or specialise in a clinical specialty. Nurses commonly undertake diplomas, first and second level degrees and PhDs while others develop specialty skills such district nursing or community practitioner/health visiting and work in primary care or the community. This is vastly different from the previous era, where, on qualification, nurses worked their way up through the hierarchy of the ward, from staff nurse to senior staff nurse and then sister. Nurses are now moving away from this traditional route, accessing a range of courses available to them at higher education institutes across the country. Online and distance learning packages are flourishing to meet the demand of time-poor qualified students who combine studying with a substantial clinical and managerial workload.

In 2004 the Agenda for Change was introduced replacing the Whitely Council, which dealt with pay and grading for all NHS staff (Department of Health, 2004a, b). The Agenda for Change, in conjunction with the NHS Job Evaluation Scheme, matches each member of staff with an appropriate pay band, directly related to their role against the Knowledge and Skills Framework (KSF) (Department of Health, 2004c). This is then evaluated locally at an annual review. There are nine successive bands with a total of 56 pay points. As staff progress through their career they pass through a number of "gateway" points in each pay band, with 5% of staff contesting their grades. Progression to another band is very difficult as complete re-evaluation of the post is required, which is a lengthy and complicated process. Many trusts introduced e-KSF as a method of uploading the outcome of annual reviews and appeals into a central database.

In 2006, the KSF was applied to all NHS jobs. Each post has a KSF post outline identifying the dimensions, levels, indicators and areas of application that are required by the post holder to undertake that role. It also prompts managers and individuals to address key areas for further development in knowledge and skill application. The KSF's aim was to be simple and easy to understand and implement and linked with the NHS Plan and to professional regulatory standards. *Table 2.3* provides an overview of the core dimensions and level descriptors.

Developments in nursing profession

As the nursing profession has developed, so new roles, such as practice nurses and nurse practitioners, have evolved to deal with specific areas of nursing responsibilities. These particular nursing specialities have been at the forefront of managing patients with urgent care needs, such as in the community and primary care settings. These roles have facilitated nurses in the autonomous management of undifferentiated patients, often with serious and long-standing health problems, in the pre-hospital setting.

Practice nursing

In 1990, the GP contract changed and GP practices were encouraged to employ practice nurses to undertake a number of clinical roles in the primary care setting. These nurses quickly became experienced and adept at treating a whole range of patients with minor injuries and illnesses and at managing and leading clinics for patients with long-term conditions, such as chronic heart disease, asthma, diabetes, etc. Many of these patients were seriously unwell, living with life-limiting diseases, such as chronic heart failure and hypertension, and admission avoidance was a key element to their clinical care; an approach latterly adopted by ECPs.

These long-term condition clinics, for which local health authorities offered financial incentives to GPs, not only improved the health of patients but also generated income for the practice. Health authorities also offered financial support for relevant nurse training and many practice nurses undertook extended roles in areas such as family planning. These clinics were supported by clinical guidelines from a number of recognised organisations, for example, guidance from the British Thoracic Society facilitated nurses in the management of patients with acute and chronic asthma. Practice nurses administered nebulised

Table 2.3. Overview of KSF core dimensions

Core dimension	Level descriptors
1. Communication	1. Communicate with a limited range of people on day-to-day matters 2. Communicate with a range of people on a range of matters 3. Develop and maintain communication with people about difficult matters and/or in difficult situations 4. Develop and maintain communication with people on complex matters, issues and ideas and/or in complex situations
2. Personal and people development	1. Contribute to own personal development 2. Develop own skills and knowledge and provide information to others to help their development 3. Develop oneself and contribute to the development of others 4. Develop oneself and others in the areas of practice
3. Health, safety and security	1. Assist in maintaining own and others' health, safety and security 2. Monitor and maintain health, safety and security of self and others 3. Promote, monitor and maintain best practice in health, safety and security 4. Maintain and develop an environment and culture that improves health, safety and security
4. Service improvement	1. Make changes in own practice and offer suggestions for improving services 2. Contribute to the improvement of services 3. Appraise, interpret and apply suggestions, recommendation and directives to improve services 4. Work in partnership with others to develop, take forward and evaluate direction, policies and strategies
5. Quality	1. Maintain the quality of own work 2. Maintain quality in own work and encourage others to do so 3. Contribute to improving quality 4. Develop a culture that improves quality
6. Equality and diversity	1. Act in ways that support equality and value diversity 2. Support equality and value diversity 3. Promote equality and value diversity 4. Develop a culture that promotes equality and diversity

bronchodilator treatment for patients suffering acute exacerbations of asthma, monitored their responses, managed their rescue therapeutic regimes and monitored them until they returned to normal respiratory status. In this way these patients avoided transfer and possible admission to hospital. This approach to care was replicated for other conditions, such as diabetes and heart disease. Prior to practice nurses, busy GPs would often have little option but to request an ambulance and transfer the patient to hospital for treatment and admission. A suitably educated and experienced practice nurse could not only manage the patient, but also be a friendly face, well-known to the patient, with full access to the medical records and able to provide continuity of care, which can break down on admission to hospital.

Many of these practice nurses also began to run the emergency sessions in GP surgeries. These sessions saw patients with largely acute, self-limiting health problems such as influenza, coughs, colds and other upper respiratory tract infections, minor injuries, urinary tract infections, patients requesting emergency contraception and so on. These "walk in" sessions, previously the domain of the GP, not only released GPs to manage more seriously unwell patients in booked appointments, but were effectively managed by the practice nurses, particularly those with additional non-medical prescribing rights.

Following publication of the Crown Report (Department of Health, 1999), practice nurses began to develop their autonomy by formalising the common and time-consuming practice of waiting patiently outside a GP's surgery door for a signature on a prescription for a medication that had often been recommended by the nurse in the first place. This move offered greater access to care for patients with long-term conditions.

Nurse practitioners

Such profound change in the advancement of primary care nursing required an equally profound change to the educational framework for these new pioneers of practice. The champion of change came in the form of Barbara Stilwell who studied the role and education of the nurse practitioner in the United States and brought the concept to the UK. The first diploma level course, delivered at the Institute of Advanced Nurse Education at the RCN in London, was predominantly accessed by primary and community-based nurses who were managing patients with a range of often complex conditions in clinics within their GP practices – and they made for avid students. Many of Barbara Stilwell's early alumni formed the basis of the advanced nurse practice we see today.

The NHS Primary Care Act (Department of Health, 1997) introduced the "first wave" of pilot schemes that set out to test different models of personal medical services aimed at providing greater flexibility in primary care provision. A number of these pilot schemes were run by GPs, others by nurses, who led teams of other healthcare professionals such as district nurses, health visitors, midwives and mental health personnel (Gardner, 1998). Such schemes provided opportunities for research and most patients were unaware that nurses were actually running the service, which was found to be both safe and effective (Chapple and Macdonald, 1999).

Some nurse practitioners worked in walk-in centres that provided a complementary service for primary care and emergency departments, managing effectively patients with a range of minor health issues (Lewis, 2001; Salisbury et al, 2002). Others developed their clinical expertise, working with medical teams in areas such as endoscopy, dermatology and cardiac surgery. The barriers between medicine and nursing were becoming increasing blurred and on the whole, this was accepted and welcomed by patients and medical colleagues.

Many of the nurse practitioner roles originated in primary care, based in community and primary care centres, managing a range of patients who may have either attended their GP or the emergency department. *Table 2.2* provides some examples of the clinical remit of these nurse practitioners. The first nurse practitioners were pioneers who pushed the boundaries of autonomous practice further than ever. They were a first point of contact for many patients who were unable to secure a GP appointment or felt unable to endure the often inevitable prolonged wait in an emergency department.

Nurse prescribing

One of the key developments to support advanced nursing practice is that of non-medical prescribing. Following publication of the Crown Report (Department of Health, 1999), which reviewed the prescribing, supply and administration of medicines, nurses were empowered to formally prescribe medication to patients. This was revolutionary at the time, as this permitted many key nurses to prescribe a range of medications to patients presenting as emergencies and those with long-term conditions.

For example, in asthma, a practice nurse would now have the ability to prescribe all the medications the patient required, such as nebulisers and steroid treatment. In the "walk in" or emergency clinics, practice nurses were now able to prescribe a range of antibiotics and analgesics for patients with a range of commonly presenting conditions, which also helped to reduce emergency department attendance.

Non-medical prescribing

Nurse prescribing began in the early 1990s and was initially limited to nurses with "community" qualifications, such as health visitors and district nurses. A review of the prescribing, supply and administration of medicines was conducted by a seminal report (Department of Health, 1999). The supply and administration of medicines was permitted under group protocols that were specific instructions developed by doctors and pharmacists for the supply or administration of named medicines by a number of healthcare practitioners, particularly nurses.

The Department of Health's NHS Plan (2000) and its *High quality care for all* document (2008) highlighted the need to organise and deliver services around the needs of patients, their families and carers. Part of this approach incorporated changes to support non-medical prescribing. Historically, this was limited to a small group of community-qualified nurses, however the new approach aimed to empower suitably and appropriately qualified healthcare professionals to prescribe a range of medications (see *Table 2.4*). Relevant academic programmes at postgraduate level were developed to support many of these advanced clinicians, outlined in *Table 2.2,* necessitating the issue of prescription-only medications (PoMs) to support their roles, following examination and management of a range of conditions. Subsequently the *Nurse Prescribers Formulary for Community Practitioners* (NPF) was released outlining those medications that nurse prescribers were able to prescribe. It is an adjunct of the *British National Formulary* (BNF) and is published by the British Medical Association and the Royal Pharmaceutical Society of Great Britain in association with the Community Practitioners' and Health Visitors' Association and the RCN. The Nursing and Midwifery Council has also published standards for practice on supplying, administration, dispensing and storage of medicines (NMC, 2008d).

The *High quality care for all: Making the connections* (Department of Health, 2009b) report further outlined how service improvements and efficiencies could be achieved by improving patient access to medicine. These examples include nurse prescribing in diabetic, hyperlipidaemia and hypertension services. For instance, patients with chronic obstructive pulmonary disease (COPD) can be treated by community heart failure nurses who can initiate and titrate medications thereby reducing hospital admissions for this patient group. The COPD guidelines published by the National Institute for Health and Clinical Excellence (NICE) outline the evidence-based rationale for managing COPD, including therapeutic management strategies, early assessment and referral advice (NICE, 2004). These guidelines are multi-professional and therefore applicable to both nurses and paramedics.

Supplementary and independent prescribing

There are currently over 49000 nurses who are registered to prescribe medicines, either as supplementary or independent nurse prescribers against professional and regulatory standards (NMC, 2006; 2008c). A total of 54 higher education institutes currently deliver a non-medical prescribing programme at a range of academic levels across the UK. These programmes permit nurses to prescribe

Table 2.4. Examples of Patient Group Directions used by paramedic and nurse practitioners

Drug	Dose	Indications
Antimicrobials		
Aciclovir	200mg and 800mg tablets	Varicella zoster
Amoxicillin	250mg and 500mg capsules 125mg/1.25ml suspension	Chest infections, otitis media
Co-amoxiclav	250/125 (amoxicillin 250mg and clavulanic acid tablets 125/31) (amoxicillin 125mg and clavulanic acid tablets 31.25mg)	Animal/human bites Alterative treatment to trimethoprim for urinary tract infections
Chloramphenicol	1% ointment	Superficial ocular infection
Erythromycin	250mg tablets 125mg/5ml suspension	Tonsillitis, otitis media, minor wounds, sinusitis, animal/human bites, chest infections
Flucloxacillin	250mg and 500mg capsules, 250mg/5ml syrup	Impetigo, otitis externa, cellulitis, pneumonia, wound prophylaxis
Metronidazole	400mg tablets, 200mg/5ml suspension	Prophylaxis of animal/ human bites (in conjunction with erythromycin)
Penicillin V	250mg tablets, 125mg/5ml and 250mg/5ml	Tonsillitis, pharyngitis, prophylaxis for wound infections (in conjunction with flucloxacillin)
Trimethoprim	200mg tablets	Uncomplicated urinary tract infections
Analgesics		
Co-codamol 8/500	Codeine phosphate 8mg and paracetamol 500mg tablets	Mild to moderate pain
Ibuprofen	200mg coated tablets, 100mg/5ml suspension	Mild to moderate pain, pyrexia
Paracetamol	500mg tablets, 125mg/5ml and 250mg/5ml suspension	Mild to moderate pain, pyrexia
Diclofenac sodium	50mg tablets, 100mg suppositories	Pain and inflammation associated with musculoskeletal conditions, gout, acute post-operative pain

Table 2.4 cont/

Table 2.4 cont/		
Gastrointestinal agents		
Prochlorperazine	5mg tablets	Nausea and vomiting
Gaviscon	Sodium alginate 500mg and potassium bicarbonate 100mg/5ml	Heartburn, gastro-oesophageal reflux, dyspepsia, epigastric discomfort
Glycerin	1gram suppositories	Constipation
Oral rehydration salts	Dioralyte powder sachets	Replacement for fluid/electrolyte loss after acute diarrhoea
Ranitidine hydrochloride	150mg tablets	Symptomatic relief of gastro-oesophageal reflux disease, chronic episodic dyspepsia, epigastric or retrosternal pain, occasionally administered with non-steroidal anti-inflammatory drugs
Respiratory agents		
Prednisolone	5mg tablets (enteric coated and soluble)	Acute asthma, exacerbation of COPD
Salbutamol	100µg aerosol inhaler	Acute exacerbation of asthma, symptomatic relief in acute exacerbation of COPD
Miscellaneous		
Chlorphenamine maleate	4mg tablets, 2mg/5ml oral solution	Symptomatic relief of hay fever and urticaria
Diazepam (refer to JRCALC guidelines for rectal use)	2mg tablets	Muscle spasm, anxiety, distress, insomnia
Fluorescein sodium	1% drops	Detection of ophthalmic foreign bodies, corneal ulcers, abrasions and burns

from an NPF against either Patient Specific Directions (PSDs) or Patient Group Directions (PGDs).

PSDs are individual written instructions from an independent prescriber for the supply or administration of medication for an individual patient, similar to a doctor's prescription. This is invaluable, for example, for advanced practitioners working in out-of-hours services with primary care organisations, managing patients with "minor" illnesses or patients attending "Minors" in an emergency department. PGDs are written instructions for a group of patients with a particular clinical condition, who are not specifically individually identified. This is useful for practice nurses and other disease-specific nurse practitioners who manage long-term conditions as it means they can supply and/or administer directly to a patient without the need for a prescription if the patient meets the criteria.

There are some excellent resources available for non-medical prescribers, particular from the National Prescribing Centre (NPC), which provides advice on PGDs and the administration and storage of medicines (NPC, 2009). In practice, the majority of non-medical prescribing programmes often combine both supplementary and independent prescribing through offering students an additional two to three days of study. This flexibility is useful, providing practitioners with an option of ensuring they have the greatest efficacy in managing a range of patients whilst maximising use of their release time from practice. A number of academic programmes are also available for first level registered nurses and midwives, who are able to study at Level 3 (6) following 3 years of post-qualification experience.

The Health and Social Care Act (Office of Public Sector Information, 2001b) designated new categories of prescribers and amended the Prescription Only Medicines Order and Supplementary Prescribing (previously referred to as Dependent Prescribing) for registered nurses, midwives and pharmacists. This is a voluntary prescribing partnership between the independent prescriber (who can be a doctor or dentist) and supplementary prescriber (e.g. nurse or healthcare practitioner) for the implementation of an agreed patient-specific clinical management plan (Department of Health, 2006a).

The legal criteria for supplementary prescribing include the prior agreement to the clinical management plan by both doctor and supplementary prescriber, an agreement that must be recorded. Both prescribers must also have access to, share and consult the same patient record.

The NPC developed a competency framework for allied health professional supplementary prescribers, with an aim of assisting higher education institutes and other professional bodies and trusts with academic programme development. The education curriculum includes consultation and decision-making skills, pharmacological principles, psychology of prescribing, monitoring techniques, legal, ethical and professional frameworks, and the importance of evidence-based practice and documentation.

In 2006, Independent Prescribing (formerly referred to as Extended Formulary Nurse Prescribing) permitted nurses to prescribe a licensed medicine, including some controlled drugs, for any medical condition that they were competent to treat. The *Medicines Matter* (Department of Health, 2006a) document was integral in developing effective prescribing, outlining key issues and updating healthcare practitioners on the developments in non-medical prescribing. All first level registered nurses, midwives, specialist community public health nurses and pharmacists can become independent prescribers. Nurses are required to have three years post-registration experience and attend a suitable academic programme.

For further examples of supplementary and independent prescribing PGDs, please refer to *Table 2.4*. Although these are examples of paramedic practitioner PGDs, they are equally relevant to paramedic and nursing practice; in fact many of the paramedic PGDs were developed from existing nurse and allied health professional PGDs.

Evidence to support practice

With the growth of the profession and greater standards for healthcare required by the public, the nursing profession began to introduce formal standards for patient care and clinical practice. Some of the measures to do this included introducing best practice guidelines from the professional bodies following research into clinical practice and adoption of education approaches that applied greater scientific criteria to practice, for example, evidence-based research. Whilst evidence-based medicine and nursing are well recognised, the role of evidence-based practice in urgent care is being established and is discussed in further detail below.

National Institute of Health and Clinical Excellence

The National Institute of Health and Clinical Excellence (NICE) is an independent organisation providing national, evidence-based guidance for a range of clinical conditions. All NICE guidelines are based on the best available evidence and financial efficacy of treatments; the latter generating angry responses from clinicians who felt that the methodological approach to some financial reviews was flawed.

NICE was set up partly in response to recommendations from the Bristol Royal Infirmary (BRI) Inquiry Report (2001) which was undertaken following the unexpected deaths of several children following cardiac surgery at the BRI. The Report, a result of a public inquiry undertaken from 1998–2001 focused on the deaths of babies born with congenital heart disease, who underwent complex cardiac surgery. The Report revealed that although paediatric cardiac surgery for these critically ill children was pushing forward the boundaries of clinical care, there had been a prolonged period of financial shortfall for funding this specialist care. This financial deficit resulted in a shortage of paediatric cardiologists, paediatric nurses and a lack of capital funding for buildings and equipment in the trust.

These specialised services were initially centrally funded, the aim being to limit the number of specialist units, by developing high levels of expertise in caring for children with relatively rare conditions. The service at the BRI was limited to children from birth to one year of age (although occasionally surgeons at the BRI carried out procedures on children over this upper age limit). From 1980 concerns began to be expressed at the standard of care delivered following the death of one particular child during surgery. Subsequently two cardiac surgeons were dismissed and conditions were applied to a third surgeon by the General Medical Council (GMC). This led to the Inquiry and its disturbing findings (Department of Health, 2002)

The Inquiry highlighted an organisational failure to communicate, a lack of leadership, paternalism and a "club culture" that essentially failed to put patients at the centre of care. Particularly alarming was the lack of performance evaluation in the NHS and the lack of assessment of the quality of care and lines of responsibility. Between 1991 and 1995 just over 30 children aged under a year died following cardiac surgery, more than double the national average for this type of surgery.

The Inquiry subsequently made almost 200 recommendations pertaining to a number of areas including the competence of HCPs, the maintenance of skills of hospital consultants through regular appraisals and CPD and steps to prevent surgeons from introducing new and invalidated techniques without any form of notification or approval. A key recommendation was the introduction of the appropriate standards of care through the development of NICE as an independent body to coordinate all actions relating to setting standards and issuing national clinical guidelines.

In essence, NICE rose from the ashes of the BRI Inquiry. NICE has a number of functions, including providing guidance on patient safety in the NHS, and its Centre for Public Health Excellence develops guidance on the promotion of good health and prevention of ill health.

NICE publishes a range of evidence-based clinical guidelines pertaining to a whole range of conditions. Most guidelines are welcomed and provide a framework for clinical practice based on the best available evidence with updates every four years. However, a number of NICE guidelines have proved controversial.

In 2003, NICE published a head injury guideline (partially updated in 2007) (NICE, 2007) that had important implications for urgent care. The guideline made recommendations for the triage, assessment, investigation and early management of head injuries focused on the "clinically important brain injury". One key recommendation suggested that patients presenting with a head injury with a Glasgow Coma Scale (GCS) score of <13 on initial assessment in the emergency department (less than 1.5–2 hours post-injury) or with a suspected skull fracture, seizure or vomiting, should receive a computerised tomography (CT) scan within one hour; the guideline essentially recommending that CT scans should replace the traditional skull x-ray in the management of head injured patients.

A number of subsequent studies suggested that implementing the NICE

41

head injury guideline would incur increased financial expense for the hospital and increased exposure to radiation for the patient (Shavrat et al, 2006). The cost would prove prohibitive, particularly in hospitals where CT access was limited and where admission for observation was effectively cheaper (Sultan et al, 2004). Other studies have argued against this point, suggesting that the increased cost of the CT scan (by two to fivefold in some instances) outweighs the benefits for patient care and the cost of admission (Hassan et al, 2005).

Other NICE resources include the *Emergency Services Current Awareness Update*; a bi-monthly newsletter providing a summary of current information to support and promote evidence-based practice in pre-hospital, ambulance and the emergency services. The Update, which covers recent research, news, best practice and policy issues, was commissioned by the National Ambulance Research Steering Group and comprises research from ambulance trusts in England and Wales with that of other experts and groups supporting pre-hospital research. The aim of the group is to support the strategic development of ambulance and pre-hospital research.

One of the most useful services that NICE provides is the NHS Evidence web-based service providing free access to high quality clinical and non-clinical information related to health and social care. Aimed at healthcare professionals and the public, NHS Evidence also provides access to subscription journals through the NHS Athens system. The most appropriate section for readers of this book is the Emergency and Urgent Care Specialist Library that hosts links to the latest Cochrane Library collection and also the latest Clinical Knowledge Summaries. The latter provide a useful source of clinical knowledge regarding common conditions managed in primary and/or urgent care. These summaries contain evidence-based information aimed at supporting healthcare professionals in their decision-making in clinical care. Each topic covers clinical presentations, management and prescribing information and advice for patients. In addition, a monthly newsletter, *Eyes on Evidence*, allows interested subscribers to keep updated on any new evidence.

Evidence-based medicine

Evidence-based medicine (EBM) aims to apply the best available evidence gained from scientific studies to support medical decision-making, assisting practitioners in assessing the risk–benefits associated with a variety of treatments. David Sackett was one of the first physicians to introduce EBM into the UK in the mid-1990s. His work in North America led him to conclude that the majority of clinical care was delivered according to the preference of the physician and not necessarily on the latest research – the BRI Inquiry being a classic example of such practice. In a much-quoted Editorial in the *British Medical Journal*, Sackett sought to explain the philosophy of EBM, defining it as "the conscientious, explicit, and judicious use of current best evidence in making decisions about the care of individual patients" (Sackett et al, 1996: 71).

EBM has its origins in mid-19th century Paris and is the integration of practitioners' clinical expertise and the best available, external clinical evidence from systematic research. Individual clinical expertise, acquired from years of clinical experience and practice, is the proficiency and judgement of the individual clinician. This expertise results in an effective and efficient diagnosis, combined with the thoughtful and compassionate understanding of the individual patient's condition and preference in decisions regarding care.

However EBM had its dissenters (Grahame-Smith, 1995). Criticism ranged from EBM being "old hat" to it being a dangerous innovation, "perpetrated by the arrogant to serve cost cutters and suppress clinical freedom" (Sackett et al, 1996: 72). *The Lancet* published an anonymous editorial liking EBM to an "attack...from within its own ranks" and lambasted the introduction of the *Evidence Based Medicine* journal grandly referring to it as the "EBM élite".

EBM is not, "cookbook medicine". It requires a triangulated approach that integrates clinical expertise, external evidence and also the often overlooked fact that patient choice and views are to be incorporated into any clinical decisions made. The fear that external evidence would replace individual clinical expertise was central to early arguments against EBM. However the subsequent evidence-based guidelines are simply that it should act as a guide to the practitioner, to assist in decision making and to ensure the suggested treatment and/or management complements the individual patient's clinical condition and preferences. It does appear extraordinary, reviewing some of the earlier disquiet in the literature today, of the arguments against EBM as it is currently implicit in everyday practice. One of the key elements that Sackett and his colleagues stressed was that central to EBM was learning – that practitioners could (and indeed should) use the implementation of EBM with teaching; thereby encouraging students to learn, whatever their discipline. Despite all the skepticism, EBM has continued to evolve, adapt and is alive and well today.

Since the introduction of EBM, a more generic approach has developed called evidence-based healthcare (EBH). This is defined as:

> *...the conscientious use of current best evidence in making decisions about the care of individual patients or the delivery of health services.*
>
> (Cochrane, 1999)

EBH also includes the consideration of potential for harm from exposure to particular agents, accuracy of diagnostic tests, and the predictive power of prognostic factors. One notable difference from EBM is that EBH should be undertaken in consultation with the patient, rather than just for the patient (Gray, 1997).

Evidence-based nursing (EBN)

Not to be outdone, EBN has also gathered strength in the UK, generating a great deal of interest. Implementing the outcomes of nursing research has historically been limited for a range of reasons, including restrictions being occasionally placed on nurses wishing to adopt findings, and nurses not fully understanding or believing research (Hunt, 1996). A study by the Centre for Evidence-Based Nursing at the University of York focused on nursing in the acute care setting and set out to clarify what EBN meant. This study by Thompson et al (2002) identified a number of elements on which nurses' clinical decision making was based, see *Figure 2.1*. The study also suggested that nurses did not always possess the required knowledge and skills to make effective use of the available research. Learning the skills of EBN, such as literature searching and appraisal were key, and without formal, supporting education in these basic skills many nurses are unable to maximise the opportunities afforded by initiatives such as NHS Evidence.

Nurses currently play a key role in the interpretation and implementation of research, specifically nurses in senior clinical positions, such as clinical nurse specialists and consultant nurses. Such nurses are clinical leaders and change agents in their own right. This role specialisation, increasingly common in nursing practice, is beginning to be evident in the pre-hospital and urgent care setting. For example the role of the advanced practitioner and consultant practitioner, as supported by the College of Paramedics, will hopefully support the concept of evidence-based paramedic practice in the future.

Gathering the evidence

Having the time and expertise to access, read and critically evaluate clinical evidence is challenging for even the most organised healthcare professional. Fortunately the Cochrane Collaboration provides a range of systematic reviews via the Cochrane Library, aimed at assisting practitioners to improve healthcare decision-making. The reviews are the combined results of the world's best clinical research studies and are recognised as the gold standard in EBH. This aids both practitioner and researcher in identifying evidence from a range of resources, specifically from randomised controlled trials. The Cochrane Collaboration removes uncertainly by ensuring that the assessed trials are unbiased and of high quality.

One example in urgent care is the Ottawa knee rules (OKR) which are based on a Canadian study of 750 children aged between 2 and 16 years presenting with knee injuries in an emergency department. This systematic review of such injuries accurately determines the management of knee fractures in children, concluding that use of the OKR can accurately identify fractures in children, specifically in those aged younger than 5 years. Although this was a North

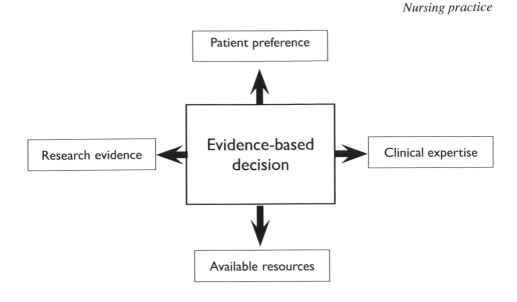

Figure 2.1. Evidence-based nursing.

American study, it has applications in the UK and can support management of knee injuries in UK emergency departments and other urgent and pre-hospital care settings. The evidence is of course multiprofessional; providing evidence for supporting both nurse and paramedic management of knee injuries and for clinical guidelines in settings with limited medical support. Application of the OKR has been found to significantly reduce the requirement to x-ray children aged over 5 years, which clearly has both positive health and financial implications (Bulloch et al, 2003).

The Cochrane Collaboration also focuses on systematic reviews that utilise explicit methodology, minimising bias in the research review process by identifying and selecting only relevant studies, and collecting and combining their data, regardless of their results. Systematic reviews are generally more consumer-friendly since they do not contain the statistical analyses of individual studies, but rather many reviewed studies are combined to produce an overall statistic, referred to as a meta-analysis. Although meta-analyses will have greater mathematical precision than their component individual studies, they will be subject to potential bias from the study selection process, and may therefore generate an accurate, but clinically misleading, outcome.

Table 2.5 outlines some examples of systematic reviews related to urgent care. These reviews are wide-ranging, some focusing on the clinical practice, whilst others review the economic feasibility of a treatment or procedure. All such reviews should be read in context, with consideration of the country of origin of the author(s), the methodological approach taken and the conclusions, before being considered for application to professional practice.

Modernising nursing careers

The document *Modernising nursing careers* (Department of Health, 2006b) reported on the outcomes of a forum of nursing leaders' of the four UK countries. It reviewed how the structure of nursing needed to change in the UK and set the direction for modernising nursing careers. Aimed predominantly at registered nurses, the report suggested that, in line with socio-economic and demographic changes in the UK, the ever-adaptable nurse would require support and development in practice, education and training, and quality and service development as well as leadership, management and supervision. As such, the four key areas that the document focused on were:

1. Development of a competent and flexible nursing workforce.
2. Updating of career pathways and career choices.
3. Preparation of nurses to lead in a changed healthcare system.
4. Modernisation of the image of nursing and nursing careers.

The report represented recognition of the range of roles that nurses undertake, frequently now supported by academic programmes up to masters and PhD level, with many nurses leading teams at senior management and executive level.

National practitioner programmes

Between 2001 and 2005, the Changing Workforce Programme, developed by the Modernisation Agency, pioneered a number of New Ways of Working teams across health and social care to deliver service improvements focusing on key workforce priorities outlined in the NHS Plan (Department of Health, 2000).

The associated National Practitioner Programmes began in 2003 and developed a number of advanced practitioners in a range of specialties, as outlined in *Appendix 2.1*. Many of these roles were available not only to nurses, but also to paramedics and operating department assistants/practitioners to develop their traditional roles to support either existing or predicted shortfalls in medical provision or to meet various national targets. The ECP and continuing care practitioner roles were early key examples of these New Ways of Working teams that had the greatest impact in urgent care. Various competency-based curriculum frameworks supported all the programmes from which higher education institutes could develop their own academic programmes.

The Darzi Review

The publication of *High Quality Care for All* (often referred to as the Darzi Review) (Department of Health, 2008) set out to launch a "new wave" of public service reforms aimed at greater utilisation of social enterprises. Interestingly

Table 2.5 Overview of systematic reviews for urgent care

Study	Objectives	Study selection	Outcomes	Comments
Giele et al (2009)	To assess effects of bracing on clinical and functional outcomes and length of stay compared with non-bracing therapies for traumatic thoracolumbar fractures.	• Systematic reviews • RCTs • Non-randomised controlled trials • Observational studies	No evidence for the effectiveness of bracing in patients admitted to hospital with traumatic thoracolumbar fractures.	Some studies excluded due to language issues, but unlikely to affect outcomes. Search dates were not reported. Assessment tool for observational studies was inappropriate and more relevant to RCTs. Small number of studies selected, but given level of evidence, conclusion are likely or be reliable.
McDermott et al (2008)	To summarise and evaluate interventions that reduce time to reperfusion in individuals with ST-segment-elevation myocardial infarction.	• Abstracts • Review of relevant full-text articles	Due to weak study design and inadequate information, specifically in terms of generalisability, there was insufficient evidence to recommend any particular intervention to reduce time to revascularisation.	The inclusion criterion was broad to include all types of interventions and search limited to English language papers, so some studies may have been missed. No apparent formal assessment of study quality, making it difficult to assess reliability of results. Most studies were low quality observational studies, which are less reliable than RCTs and therefore author's cautious conclusions are reliable.

Table 2.5/cont

Table 2.5/cont

Roberts and Mays (1997)	To assess whether, and to what extent, primary care based emergency services can substitute for the traditional hospital accident and emergency department model of emergency services.	• RCTs • Quasi-experimental studies • Controlled before-and-after studies • Retrospective studies	Access to primary care was an important influence on patient demand for accident and emergency care. The focus of substitution may be a means of providing cost-effective emergency care.	Methodological quality of systematic review was high, with extensive literature review. The authors noted the limitations of the findings.
Guo and Harstakk (2006)	The report aims to identify strategies that have been evaluated and reported in the literature and assess their effectiveness in reducing emergency department overcrowding.	Not stated	Report was a benchmark for current published research. Standardised definitions for emergency department overcrowding and other relevant terms.	None provided.

the first image in this document is that of an ECP making his way to a patient in a rural location – perhaps this was felt to typify the example of the radical changes to healthcare services that are required?

The reforms in the Darzi Review were aimed at providing locally delivered, patient-centred care based on patient need where it is required, which inevitably would lead to changes in service delivery. Primary care trusts were encouraged to set up social enterprises and many nurses have welcomed these new models of healthcare delivery, using their advanced clinical skills and expertise. Locally developed services have greater flexibility and are more responsive to community needs. Some of the examples provided in the Darzi Review are in the pre-hospital or urgent care setting, such as acute care in specialised trauma centres for major trauma, myocardial infarction and stroke, supported by skilled ambulance practitioners. Children's clinical pathways are to be provided in settings closer to the child's home, such as schools and other child centres. Mental health services are also to be delivered differently; from community rather than a traditional hospital or outpatient/clinic setting.

Other suggested changes in urgent need are those of improved patient information for accessing urgent care, such as a three-digit telephone number to assist people in finding the right service to meet urgent care needs, for example late-night pharmacies or emergency dentists. Unlocking talents of existing clinicians, such as paramedics, in a team approach to care, was considered essential for high quality clinical care. Whilst the Darzi Review does not refer specifically to advanced paramedic roles such as the paramedic practitioner, utilising the advanced skills and competencies of such individuals will inevitably be one of the key elements in the successful delivery and implementation of the Review's proposals. For too long, the ambulance service has worked in isolation from NHS trusts, particularly primary care trusts, and some of the key community and primary care services. It would be very refreshing to witness some of the proposed "joined-up thinking" becoming a reality, ensuring that the paramedic's expertise is more effectively utilised.

Nursing today

Currently there are 670 000 registered nurses in the UK working in four different branches. The majority are adult nurses (397 000), followed by mental health nurses (61 000), children's nurses (19 000) and learning disabilities nurses (14 000).

Nursing roles have changed and developed, particularly within associated medical specialities, such as infection control and public health. Nurses now have specific disease-focused roles such as respiratory and cardiac nurse specialists. The latter have evolved from the generic nurse practitioners and nurse consultants. Some nurses work in an independent capacity developing social enterprise initiatives, which are businesses set up to tackle social and environmental needs, many of which are related to health.

References

Bradshaw A (1997) Defining 'competency' in nursing (Part 1): A policy review. *Journal of Clinical Nursing* **6**(5): 347–54

Bradshaw A (1998) Defining 'competency' in nursing (Part 11): An analytical review. *Journal of Clinical Nursing* **6**(2): 103–111

Bradshaw A, Merriman C (2008) Nursing competence 10 years on: fit for practice and purpose yet? *Journal of Clinical Nursing* **17**(10): 1263–9

Bristol Royal Infirmary Inquiry (2001) T*he Report of the Public Inquiry into children's heart surgery at the Bristol Royal Infirmary 1984–1995*. London: HMSO

Bulloch B, Neto G, Plint A, Lim R, Lidman P, Reed M, Nijssen-Jordan C, Tenenbein M, Klassen TP (2003) The Ottawa Knee Rules accurately identified fractures in children with knee injures. *Annals of Emergency Medicine* **42**(1): 48–55

Chapple A, Macdonald W (1999) A nurse-led pilot scheme: The patient's perspective. *Primary Health Care* **19**(2): 16–17

Cochrane AL (1999) *Random reflections on health services*. London: Royal Society of Medicine Press

Department of Health (1946) *National Health Service Act*. London: HMSO

Department of Health (1997) *National Health Service (Primary Care) Act 1997*. London: HMSO

Department of Health (1999) *Review of prescribing, supply and administration of medicines: Final report. (Crown Report)* London: HMSO

Department of Health (2000) *The NHS Plan. A plan for investment. A plan for reform*. London: HMSO

Department of Health (2002) *Learning from Bristol. The Department of Health's response to the Report of the Public Inquiry into children's heart surgery at the Bristol Royal Infirmary 1984–1995*. London: HMSO

Department of Health (2004a) *Agenda for Change – Final agreement*. London: HMSO

Department of Health (2004b) *NHS Job Evaluation Handbook* (2nd Edn). London: HMSO

Department of Health (2004c) *Overview of the NHS KSF*. London: HMSO

Department of Health (2005) *Taking healthcare to the patient – Transforming NHS ambulance services*. London: HMSO

Department of Health (2006a) *Medicines Matter*. London: HMSO

Department of Health (2006b) *Modernising nursing careers – setting the direction*. London: HMSO

Department of Health (2008) *High quality care for all. NHS next stage review*. Final Report. London: HMSO

Department of Health (2009a) *NHS Direct Annual Report 2008/9*. London: HMSO

Department of Health (2009b) *High quality care for all: Making the connections*. London: HMSO

Gardner L (1998) Nurse-led primary care act pilot schemes: Threat or opportunity? *Nursing Times* **94**(27): 52–3

Grahame-Smith D (1995) Evidence based medicine: Socratic dissent. *British Medical Journal* **310**(6986): 1126–7

Gray JAM (1997) *Evidence-based healthcare: How to make health policy and management decisions*. London: Churchill Livingstone

Hassan Z, Smith M, Littlewood S, Bouamra O, Hughes D, Biggin C, Amos K, Mendelow AD, Lecky F (2005) Head injuries: A study evaluating the impact of the NICE head injury guidelines. *Emergency Medicine Journal* **22**(12): 845–9

Heyworth J (2001) The NHS Plan – the sound of cavalry or zebras. *Emergency Medicine Journal* **18**(1): 1–2

Hunt JM (1996) Guest Editorial. *Journal of Advanced Nursing* **23**(3): 423–5

Lewis R (2001) *Nurse-led primary care: Learning from PMS pilots*. London: Kings Fund

Mayor S (2000) Health watchdog criticises NHS helpline. *British Medical Journal* **321**: 4010

Munro J, Nicholl J, O'Cathain A, Knowles E (2000) Impact of NHS Direct in demand for immediate care: Observational study. *British Medical Journal*. **321**(7254): 150–3

National Institute for Health and Clinical Excellence (2004) *Chronic obstructive pulmonary disease: Management of chronic obstructive pulmonary disease in adults in primary and secondary care*. London: NICE

National Institute for Health and Clinical Excellence (2007) *Head injury: Triage, assessment, investigation and early management of head injury in infants, children and adults*. London: NICE

National Prescribing Centre (2009) *Patient Group Directions – December 2009*. Liverpool: NPC

Nightingale F (1969) *Notes on nursing: What it is and what it is not*. New York: Dover Publications

Nursing and Midwifery Council (2004) *Standards of proficiency for pre-registration nursing education*. London: NMC

Nursing and Midwifery Council (2006) *Standards of proficiency for nurse and midwife prescribers*. London: NMC

Nursing and Midwifery Council (2008a) *The Code - Standards of conduct, performance and ethics for nurses and midwives*. London: NMC

Nursing and Midwifery Council (2008b) *The PREP Handbook*. London: NMC

Nursing and Midwifery Council (2008c) *Statistical analysis of the Register 1 April 2007 to 31 March 2008*. London: NMC

Nursing and Midwifery Council (2008d) *Standards for Medicines Management*. London: NMC

Office of Public Sector Information (2001a) *Nursing and Midwifery Order 2001*. London: TSO.

Office of Public Sector Information (2001b) *Health and Social Care Act 2001*. London: TSO

Peacock PJ, Peacock JL, Victor CR, Chazot C (2005) Changes in the emergency workload of the London Ambulance Service between 1989 and 1999. *Emergency Medicine Journal* **22**(1): 56–9

Quality Assurance Agency (2008) *Framework for higher education qualifications in England, Wales and Northern Ireland*. Gloucester: QAA

Sackett D, Rosenberg WMC, Muir Gray JA, Haynes RB, Scott Richardson W (1996) Evidence-based medicine: What it is and what it isn't. *British Medical Journal* **312** (7023): 71–2

Salisbury C, Chalder M, Scott TM, Pope C, Moore L (2002) What is the role of walk-in centres in the NHS? *British Medical Journal* **324**(7334): 399–402

Shavrat BP, Huseyin TS, Hynes KA (2006) NICE guideline for the management of head injury: An audit demonstrating its impact on a district general hospital, with a cost analysis for England and Wales. *Emergency Medicine Journal* **23**(2): 109–13

Sultan HY, Boyle A, Pereira M, Antoun N, Maimaris C (2004) Application of the Canadian CT head rules in managing minor head injuries in a UK emergency department: Implications for the implementation of the NICE guidelines. *Emergency Medicine Journal* **21**(4): 420–5

Thompson C, McCaughan D, Cullum N, Sheldon TR (2002) Nursing, the value of research in clinical decision making. *Nursing Times* **98**(42): 30–4

Section 1: Useful Resources/Websites

Allied Health Profession Leadership Challenges Project
   http://www.youtube.com/watch?v=MBeSLZdC3R0&feature=channel
British National Formulary
   http://bnf.org/bnf/index.htm
Centre for Reviews and Dissemination
   http://www.york.ac.uk/inst/crd/
Health Quality Improvement Partnership – National Ambulance Clinical
   Audit Steering Group
   http://www.hqip.org.uk/national-ambulance-clinical-audit-steering-group
National Institute for Health Research
   http://www.nihr.ac.uk/Pages/default.aspx
NHS Evidence – emergency and urgent care
   http://www.library.nhs.uk/emergency/
Nurse Prescribers Formulary
   http://bnf.org/bnf/extra/current/450057.htm

Journals
British Journal of Nursing
   http://www.britishjournalofnursing.com
Emergency Medicine Journal
   http://Emergency Medicine Journal.British Medical Journal.com/
Evidence-based Nursing
   http://ebn.British Medical Journal.com/info/about.dtl
JEMS
   http://www.jems.com/
Journal of Paramedic Practice
   http://www.paramedicpractice.com
Primary Health Care Journal
   http://primaryhealthcare.rcnpublishing.co.uk/

Appendix 2.1

New Ways of Working programmes

New Ways of Working in emergency care

Emergency Care Practitioners

Individuals and examples of care

- Nurses and paramedics
- Roadside to emergency department
- Managing patients at home

Potential impact on health service

- Reducing transfer to emergency department
- Meeting 4-hour emergency department trolley waits
- Reducing impact on primary care out of hours
- Competence and Curriculum Framework for the ECP (Skills for Health, 2007a)
- *Emergency Care Practitioners Report* (Department of Health, 2004)

New Ways of Working in Surgery

Surgical Care Practitioners

Individuals and examples of care

- Pre-, intra- and postoperative care
- Diagnostic and surgical interventions
- A non-medical practitioner, working in clinical practice as a member of the extended surgical team, who performs surgical intervention, pre-operative and postoperative care under the direction and supervision of a consultant surgeon

Potential impact on health service

- To bring into the mainstream
- Managing pre- and postoperative care of patients
- Working in day care units
- Undertaking a range of investigative procedures, e.g. sigmoidoscopy, colonoscopy
- Reducing waiting lists
- *Competence and Curriculum Framework* document (Department of Health, 2005)

Peri-operative Specialist Practitioners

Individuals and examples of care

- Pre- and postoperative care (ward/clinic only)
- A non-medical practitioner, working at an advanced level in clinical

practice ensuring continuity of patient care within pre-operative and post-operative settings and supervised by a consultant surgeon working as a permanent member of the extended surgical team.

Potential impact on health service

- The curriculum framework for the perioperative specialist practitioner.
- Under the direction of a consultant surgeon, PSPs may participate in:
  - pre-operative assessment and physical examination
  - preparing patients for surgery including venepuncture and cannulation, male and female catheterisation, arterial blood sampling
  - performing technical procedures according to their scope of practice
  - facilitating the continuity of care of patients
  - providing pre- and postoperative investigations as part of the multidisciplinary team
  - liaising with medical, theatre, ward and clerical staff on relevant issues, such as theatre lists, to support coherent service provision
  - postoperative care, including wound assessment, initial treatment and identification of surgical problems and complications; and
  - evaluating care, including the discharge process and follow-up arrangements for surgical patients, within the scope of their competence and practice

Assistant Theatre Practitioners

Individuals and examples of care

- Assistant theatre practitioners are trained, non-registered healthcare professionals capable of performing circulating, scrub and, potentially, recovery support roles, which are limited by local protocol and practice.
- Work in theatre and obstetrics and gynaecology

Potential impact on health service

- Assistant theatre practitioners work as part of the perioperative obstetric team under the supervision of a registered practitioner
- Prepare instruments, trolleys and sterile supplies
- Provide skilled assistance to surgeon during surgery
- Perform swab, needle, blade and instrument count with the circulating practitioner
- Undertake scrub role for a limited range of cases

Endoscopy practitioners

Individuals and examples of care

- Nurse, physiologist, physicians' assistant

Potential impact on health service

- Reduced colonscopy waiting lists
- Potential for flexible sigmoidoscopy
- Potential impact on bowel screening

New Ways of Working in Medicine

Physicians' Assistant (previously referred to as Medical Care Practitioner)

Individuals and examples of care

- Nurses, science graduates
- A new healthcare professional who, while not a doctor, works to the medical model, with the attitudes, skills and knowledge base to deliver holistic care and treatment within the general medical and/or general practice team under defined levels of supervision

Potential impact on health service

- Increasing capacity in primary and secondary care through widening resource of healthcare practitioners
- *Competence and Curriculum Framework for the Medical Care Practitioner* (Department of Health, 2005)

New Ways of Working in Critical Care

Assistant Critical Care Practitioners

Individuals and examples of care

- The assistant critical care practitioner role is a new way of working that complements existing roles within the critical care team. The purpose of the role is to provide patient-focused care, previously undertaken by a registered practitioner, allowing the latter to focus on more complex care needs. Their core purpose is to ensure patient-centred, safe, timely, accessible, appropriate and efficient care, to support patients through critical illness, and, where appropriate, provide comfort and care to enable a dignified death
- An assistant practitioner is defined as a healthcare worker who delivers healthcare to patients and who has a level of knowledge and skill beyond that of the traditional healthcare assistant or support worker (WDC Standing Conference June 2003)

Potential impact on health service

- Development of care pathways
- Assistant critical care practitioners can have an impact within critical care units and as part of the provision of acute services. This may include intensive care and high dependency units, outreach, post-anaesthetic care units and medical assessment units
- The *National Education and Competence Framework for Assistant Critical Care Practitioner* (Department of Health, 2008)

Advanced Critical Care Practitioners

Individuals and examples of care

- Nurses in critical care units

- Small pilot project focusing on critical care paramedics
- The purpose of the advanced critical care practitioner role is to provide care that is focused on patients and their needs, save life, recognise acutely ill patients, initiate early treatment, support patients through critical illness and, where appropriate, enable a dignified death. The inclusion of advanced critical care practitioners in the team will enhance continuity and quality of care.

Potential impact on health service
- Undertake an extensive assessment of the critically ill patient, including taking a history and completing a clinical examination
- Perform or order diagnostic and therapeutic procedures
- Prescribe medications and fluids (subject to current legislation)
- Develop and manage an acute management plan and pathway for the patient
- Perform invasive interventions, advanced airway skills, vascular access and other practical skills under appropriate supervision dependent on experience
- Teach and educate patients, relatives and other members of the multi-professional team. Undertake internal and inter-hospital transfers of critically ill patients
- Develop existing roles in critical care
    - Develop role of paramedics in air ambulances
    - Reduce workload on medical/critical care teams in inter-hospital transfers
    - The *National Education and Competence Framework for Advanced Critical Care Practitioners* (Department of Health, 2008)

New Ways of Working in Anaesthesia

Anaesthesia Practitioners
Individuals and examples of care
- Either healthcare professional or science graduate who will have the ability to
    - perform duties delegated to them by their consultant anaesthetist supervisor
    - include pre- and post-operative patient assessment and care
    - administer anaesthesia and caring for the patient during surgical procedures
    - maintain anaesthesia (under direct supervision)
    - conduct the induction of and emergence from anaesthesia
- APs will also deputise for anaesthetists
- Other roles including monitoring, interpreting and acting on physiological changes

- Assisting with elective surgery waiting lists
- Development of existing roles
- http://www.dh.gov.uk/prod_consum_dh/groups/dh_digitalassets/@dh/@
  en/documents/digitalasset/dh_074708.pdf

Potential impact on health service

- Assisting with elective surgery waiting lists
- Development of existing roles
- http://www.dh.gov.uk/prod_consum_dh/groups/dh_digitalassets/@dh/@
  en/documents/digitalasset/dh_074708.pdf

Section Two

Clinical leadership

Clinical leadership encompasses a number of activities, such as clinical supervision, mentorship and reflective practice. All these activities are important in creating and sustaining a culture of clinical excellence within any organisation.

Clinical supervision and mentorship are "tools" by which practitioners can develop their own professional and clinical practice and they also support the future workforce through learning and development of students. This second section focuses on the concept of clinical leadership and provides an overview drawn from the Report of the National Steering Group on Clinical Leadership in the Ambulance Service (NHS ACEG, 2009a). Some models of clinical supervision and mentorship in relation to urgent care are presented and the difference between the two concepts is highlighted. Issues related to the assessment of students in clinical practice and the management of the struggling student are also included.

The section concludes with an overview of reflective practice. Reflective practice is becoming an increasingly common method by which to support practitioners and students, and can, when used appropriately and effectively, be a powerful learning tool.

CHAPTER 3

Clinical leadership in urgent care

Clinical leadership is a much quoted concept which is discussed and referred to in many key policy documents. However, its actual implementation and application is rather more elusive and therefore this chapter aims to describe and outline some of the defining attributes of clinical leadership.

Some of the text presented within this chapter has been adapted from the Report of the National Steering Group on Clinical Leadership in the Ambulance Service (NHS ACEG, 2009a) of which I was a member and, as such, my fellow co-authors are duly acknowledged.

This chapter outlines a proposed framework for clinical leadership for urgent care practice. It also presents an adapted transformational leadership model as a framework for practice and local implementation and provides practical examples. The principles are based on a number of documents, including the NHS Leadership Qualities Framework (NHS Institute for Innovation and Improvement, 2006) that sets the standard for outstanding leadership in the NHS. The Leadership Qualities Framework summarises the benefits of clinical leadership, which include improved clinical standards and governance within organisations, greater support for organisations to meet core standards set by Standards for Better Health, the NHS Litigation Authority and the Healthcare Commission Annual Assessment and also provides the infrastructure to reduce and manage clinical risk and reduce litigation.

There is an increased need for appropriate and timely preparation for clinical leadership (Cook and Leathard, 2004). A number of current programmes involve generic, decontextualised learning and often fail to address the unique problems encountered within urgent care settings as these techniques are drawn from the business world. Some clinical leadership programmes overcome these barriers; however they are generally aimed at healthcare professionals already in a leadership post, which is arguably too late and potentially frustrating for those new to the leadership role.

Clinical leadership should be implicit to advanced practitioners – something that all professionals should be striving towards – not just a disparate and alienated concept that individuals feel is unachievable or irrelevant to their practice. However to be a clinical leader individuals need to have the knowledge, skills and attributes to lead. The relevant professional and regulatory bodies, such as the Health Professions Council, the College of Paramedics and the

Nursing and Midwifery Council, set standards for professional activity that incorporate best practice and standards for conduct, performance and ethical dimensions to which practitioners are required to adhere and which form the basis of clinical leadership.

What is clinical leadership?

Clinical leadership can be defined as "the ability to both create and sustain an organisational culture of excellence through continual development and improvement" (Pintar et al 2007: 115). Clinical leadership is a method by which practitioners influence others to set standards, accomplish objectives, and direct their organisation to greater levels of cohesion. Effective leadership is one of the key elements in modernising today's health service and plays an increasingly important role in the NHS. The importance of clinical leadership was initially emphasised in the document *Making a Difference* (Department of Health, 1999) and the NHS Plan (Department of Health, 2000). Similarly, the NHS Institute for Innovation and Improvement's (2006) stated mission is to improve health outcomes and quality of care. This establishes the framework for clinical leadership practice within the NHS. The document *Shifting the Balance of Power* (Department of Health, 2002) also outlines a number of elements for outstanding leadership in the NHS such as:

- Personal development
- Board development
- Leadership profiling for recruitment and selection
- Career mapping
- Succession planning
- Connecting leadership capability.

The benefits of clinical leadership to an organisation are on a number of levels. At an organisational level, staff are better equipped to adapt and thrive in response to an ever-changing environment, particularly in the urgent care setting. On an individual level, there are benefits in terms of personal development and improvement in knowledge and skills. On a patient level, the concept of a clinically-led learning organisation would suggest a greater responsiveness to patient needs, as well as an improved ability to meet those needs, and improved care for patients (Timpson, 1998).

The operating framework for the NHS in England 2009/10 (Department of Health, 2008) outlined the commitment of the NHS to introduce talent and leadership initiatives at regional levels in order to support leadership, capacity and capability at a local level. It announced plans for a new National Leadership Council that would nurture the future generation of NHS leaders (Dawson et al, 2009). The Council will focus on standards and will be involved in intelligence and evidence gathering, setting standards and taking a strategic role in commissioning leadership development programmes.

Clinical leaders

Perhaps the key to successful clinical leadership are the clinical leaders themselves. Defining a clinical leader can be challenging, but it has been suggested that a clinical leader is "an expert clinician, involved in providing clinical care that continuously improves care through influencing others" (Cook, 2001: 39).

Clinical leaders are generally identified by a number of key characteristics which include knowledge, skills and attributes.

Knowledge

Clinically experienced practitioners develop judgement and a sense of salience (or awareness) of their environment as they become more experienced and accomplished practitioners (Benner, 2001).

Required knowledge varies according to profession. The Quality Assurance Agency's Subject Benchmark Statements for nursing and paramedic science (Quality Assurance Agency, 2001, 2004) outline the generic statements that apply to all practitioners and against which higher education institution programmes are measured. (The majority of registerable academic nursing programmes are delivered by higher education institutions.)

Paramedics have traditionally been taught by on-the-job or in-house training. However there is a shift towards university paramedic education in the UK. The development of the Foundation Degree, Diploma and first level degree qualifications provides a theoretical basis for clinical practice, and they increasingly incorporate clinical leadership. In addition, the current Joint Royal Colleges Ambulance Liaison Committee Guidelines (2006) form the basis of clinical protocols and guidelines in the NHS ambulance service thereby further informing the practitioner of evidence-based practice. The revised College of Paramedics/British Paramedic Association Career Framework (2008) outlines specific roles for ambulance clinicians based on the Skills for Health Career Framework. These roles are related to the proposed clinical leadership ladder (discussed later in this chapter) that identifies the various roles that are becoming increasingly supported by higher education institution programmes.

Skills

The Health Professions Council has identified a number of generic and specific skills in their various Standards of Proficiency for each allied healthcare profession. In their Standards for Paramedics (Health Professions Council,

2007) a range of skills are identified and, similar to the Knowledge and Skills Framework (KSF) in the NHS, these skills represent a variety of levels by which healthcare professionals develop in their clinical practice (Department of Health, 2004). Adapted from nursing, the Dreyfus and Dreyfus Novice to Expert Model (Benner, 2001) is used extensively as a basis for nurses developing from student to senior/consultant roles. The concept is that skills, both practical and theoretical, are gained over time through repeated clinical experiences that shape the clinician's preconceived notions, finally leading towards expertise, or the expert practitioner. This is developed through five stages of proficiency.

It has been suggested (NHS ACEG, 2009b) that the NHS should consider funding a research programme to develop the "productive ambulance team" concept further where "self-managing teams" make maximum use of systems, procedures, and clinical and performance information to acquire skills that deliver enhanced performance, productivity and staff satisfaction.

Attributes

Research undertaken by Cook and Leathard (2004) identified six attributes of transformational leadership for effective clinical leaders. These were:

- Developing a shared vision
- Inspiring and communicating
- Valuing others
- Challenging and stimulating
- Developing trust
- Enabling.

As a practical example of attributes, the transformational leadership approach is one that describes how motivated professionals can perform to their full potential by influencing change in perceptions and providing a sense of direction to others (Bass and Avolio, 1990). As we have seen, clinical leaders are motivational figures, inspiring others around them to develop and progress.

Transformational leadership model

Burns (1978) initially developed the concept of transformational leadership, describing it as a process whereby an individual engages with others, creates a connection and raises levels of motivation. Transformational leadership is concerned with changing and transforming individuals by instilling faith and respect, and is concerned with ethics, values, standards and long-term goals. It aims to enable those in an organisation to lead themselves.

Table 3.1. Suggested knowledge, skills and attributes of clinical leaders working in urgent care

Knowledge
- Applied anatomy and physiology
- Pharmacological principles
- Trauma care
- Airway and circulatory management
- Ethical, legal and moral issues
- Managing acute, minor and moderate illness, and minor injury, and acute episodes in long-term conditions
- Speciality clinical areas – medicine, surgery, cardiology, respiratory medicine, gastroenterology, older patients, renal medicine, neurology, haematology, obstetrics and gynaecology, rheumatology, etc.
- Branches of nursing – paediatrics, mental health, learning disabilities
- Professional issues and accountability

Source
- IHCD training, continuing professional development (CPD) and university education programmes
- College of Paramedics/British Paramedic Association Education/Career Framework (2008)
- Paramedic Association Curriculum Guidance and Competence Framework (2008)
- Quality and Assurance Agency (2004, 2006) Nurse and Paramedic Benchmark Statement
- Nursing and Midwifery Council (2008) Standards of Conduct, Performance and Ethics
- Higher Education Institutes

Skills
- Clinical skills – emergency care assistant technician, paramedic, advanced paramedic, paramedic practitioner
- Student nurse, staff nurse, junior/senior nurse, ward manager, modern matron, nurse practitioners, consultant nurses
- Communication skills
- Behavioural skills (e.g. human and situational factors)

Source
- Skills for Health Career Framework
- Dreyfus and Dreyfus (2000); Benner (2001) Novice to Expert model of skills acquisition:
  - Novice
  - Advanced beginner
  - Competent
  - Proficient
  - Expert
- JRCALC Clinical Guidelines (2006)

Table 3.1 cont/

Table 3.1. cont/
Attributes
<ul><li>Six attributes of transformational leadership (Cook and Leathard, 2004)<ul><li>Developing a shared vision</li><li>Inspiring and communicating</li><li>Valuing others</li><li>Challenging and stimulating</li><li>Developing trust</li><li>Enabling</li></ul></li></ul>*Source*<ul><li>Health Professions Council (2008) Standards of Conduct, Performance and Ethics</li><li>NMC (2008) Code of Conduct, Performance and Ethics</li></ul>
Adapted from the Report of the National Steering Group on Clinical Leadership in the Ambulance Service (NHS ACEG, 2009a)

Transformational leadership can be used to motivate "followers" to perform to their full potential over time by influencing a change in perceptions and providing a sense of direction (Bass and Avolio, 1990). The knowledge required to motivate others is referred to as transformational knowledge or "soft" knowledge that often defies definition; sometimes referred to as "intuition" or wisdom. Transformational knowledge is often considered messy; consisting of informal or personal knowledge, arising from experience of both knowledge "in action" and "on action" (Schön, 1983). Effective clinical leaders frequently demonstrate "embodied intelligence" where they take action without being able to articulate their rationale – sometimes described as having an "understanding without a rationale". Some view this as an irrational action, involving pure guesswork, but experienced practitioners can possess intuitive judgement with a sense of salience, or awareness, of their environment (Benner, 2001; Dreyfus and Dreyfus, 2000). The key qualities of intuition are difficult to articulate and assess but are evident in many clinical leaders of today.

There is a charismatic quality in great clinical leaders that attracts and influences their "followers" and this is often concerned with their relational rather than their positional power. Most of us can probably recall a particularly inspirational individual, who may have been a clinician, supervisor or lecturer and who, although not necessarily having a position of authority, possessed a certain appeal and facilitated our development and growth as practitioners. Really good clinical leaders are often expert, frontline staff who are visionary and are able to facilitate such inspiration in others. Managing this "vision" is central to transformational leadership, providing meaning and direction to practice and uniting staff in a common purpose. One of the major constraints in developing transformational leadership in an organisation is the well-established "parental–hierarchical" stance frequently observed in the NHS, often associated with the need to avoid conflict that is often pervasive amongst leaders. Transformational leadership is also characterised by trusting and collaborative relationships between colleagues at all levels of the organisation.

Transactional leadership model

In the more conventional transactional leadership, the leader adopts a more authoritarian approach, so that the team are worked "on" as opposed to being worked "with", as in transformational leadership. It is a subtle but distinct difference, having significantly different outcomes as the latter places priority on task achievement. Johns (2003) suggested that transactional leadership is characterised by the emphasis on positional reward that sanctions types of power whereas transformational leadership is characterised more by relational and expert types of power. Such leaders were often viewed as "liberating".

Transactional leaders are often successful or effective in that they maintain stability through fulfilling their roles in relation to organisational policies and procedures and the achievement of organisational goals. Transactional leadership is based on the presumption that a practitioner is not required to be a natural leader to manage. The transactional leadership theory is defined by the fact that such a leader frequently holds a senior management position within the organisational hierarchy. Although transactional leaders frequently maintain the organisational status quo, with fixed and firm fundamental expectations, the model is often criticised for lacking a vision in the future of organisational development, particularly in relation to healthcare (Gopee, 2008).

Implementing clinical leadership in organisations

The implementation of clinical leadership will vary between organisations, however the core concepts underpinning a strategic framework are knowledge, skills and attributes that support development (see *Table 3.1*). The College of Paramedics have incorporated the Skill for Health Career Framework within their current Curriculum Guidance and Competence Framework (College of Paramedics, 2008). This guidance provides a basis on which to create a flexible career path, and acquire the necessary knowledge and skills to enable an individual member of staff with transferable, competence-based skills to progress in a direction that meets patient, service, workforce and individual needs. Developing the knowledge and skill of paramedics and nurses in urgent care is essential and should include junior and senior management. Internal promotion and succession planning offers opportunities for all staff to develop their career opportunities, and helps to progress best practice and service innovation. In essence, clinical leadership is about clinical staff at all levels being actively engaged in the continuous improvement of the quality and safety of patient services.

Limitations to practice

A fundamental issue of clinical leadership is the difficulty of applying it to clinical practice. Cook and Leathard (2004) identified four key reasons for this apparent lack of application. First, there was often no commonly agreed definition or descriptor of clinical leadership, a fundamental but frequently overlooked task. It is clearly difficult to establish a clinical leadership programme within an organisation if the underlying concept remains vague. Second, clinical leaders themselves were not required to undertake any compulsory educational preparation. Such practice may of course have changed since this study although one suspects that time restraints imposed by clinical, managerial and other activities undertaken by these individuals may prohibit any time-protected preparation. Third, where academic preparation was available, it was often uni-professional, providing little opportunity to engage with healthcare professionals from a range of clinical disciplines. Last, many of the clinical leadership programmes were reportedly "disconnected" from wider organisational strategies and strategic direction, resulting in a "silo effect" therefore potentially alienating a single directorate or team from the rest of the organisation, resulting in frustration at the failure of the concept.

Proposed clinical leadership framework

The Report of the National Steering Group on Clinical Leadership in the Ambulance Service (NHS ACEG, 2009a) proposed a Clinical Leadership Framework and identified four essential elements:

- Personal mastery
- Systems thinking
- Enabling team learning
- Developing a shared vision.

Figure 3.1 outlines the four elements for clinical leadership developed from these concepts, combined with the identified knowledge, skills and attributes outlined earlier. Each of these four elements has a number of descriptors. For example, in personal mastery, a clinical leader would need to have clinical credibility. This would suggest a senior, experienced paramedic who was respected by his/her peers and was acknowledged to have a high level of clinical capability. Such practitioners would also need to be creative and

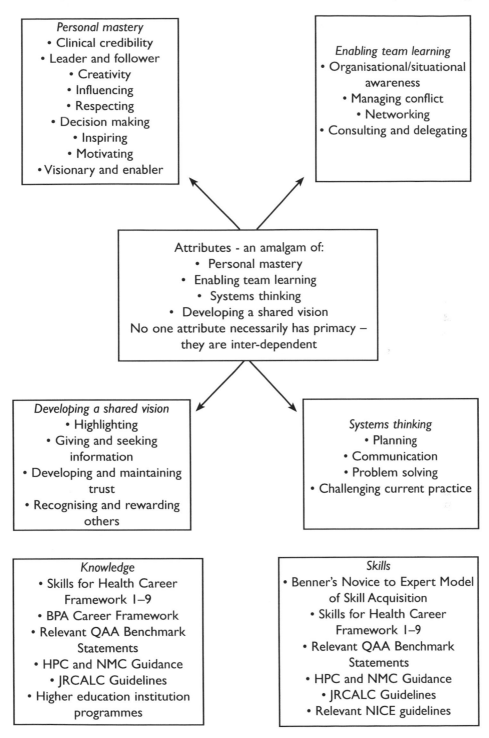

Figure 3.1. Four elements for clinical leadership.

have the ability to influence their team and ensure the team had the necessary resources to perform its role.

Clinical leadership is evolving and not all clinical leaders will necessarily have all these elements, or indeed call upon them all the time. For example, personal mastery is arguably only achieved through Masters level study, which has only recently been available to paramedics. Supporting autonomous practice is probably most important in terms of the clinical leader, since this self-motivational competency will be a driving force in this individual. Perhaps the most essential element of the role is clinical credibility and the capacity to make decisions – often rapidly and with limited resources – and also to possess a vision of the future for themselves and others. This is an example of an effective clinical leader.

The other core elements of enabling team learning, systems thinking and developing a shared vision are elements that are achieved over time, with

Table 3.2. Clinical Leadership Self-Assessment Tool

Clinical Leadership Elements	Suggested leadership examples for practice	Organisational self-assessment
Personal mastery • Clinical credibility • Problem solving processes • Leader and follower • Creativity • Influencing and respecting • Decision making • Inspiring and visionary • Motivating	• Identify existing staff to support graduate and academic students in clinical practice • Facilitate mentorship in the organisation • Develop patient assessment and history taking skills • Clinical policy influence and implementation • Are the any practice development opportunities, e.g. developing airway masterclass?	Assess against, for example: NHS Litigation Authority or clinical/key performance indicators
Developing a shared vision • Highlight and promote importance of clinical governance. • Give and seek information • Develop and maintain trust • Recognise and reward contribution of others • Clinical innovation • Professional issues and accountability	• Identify a "clinical champion" for each clinical area/station • Focus on a key clinical governance issue • Liaise with local respiratory physician, clinical nurse specialist and pharmacist to develop new care pathways • Review existing clinical guidelines • Develop a Special Interest Group in a clinical area, e.g. diabetes	Assess against, for example: National Health Service Litigation Authority or clinical/key performance indicators
		Table 3.2 cont/

Table 3.2 cont/		
Enabling team learning • Organisational/situational awareness • Managing conflict • Networking • Consulting and delegating • Building relationships within NHS organisation and wider community • Ethical, legal and moral issues	• *Provide local support and review Serious Untoward Incidents or Patient Safety Alerts* • *Collaborative working with local PCTs* • *Identify areas of shared clinical concern* • *Review informed consent guidelines*	Assess against, for example: National Health Service Litigation Authority or clinical/key performance indicators
Whole systems thinking • Planning • Communication • Problem solving • Challenging current practice	• *Initiate evidence-based practice sessions* • *Develop a clinical audit group* • *Develop a research group to review relevant qualitative and quantitative research papers* • *Review/develop clinical pathway* • *Review equipment on board ambulance*	Assess against, for example: NHS Litigation Authority or clinical performance indicators
Adapted from the Report of the National Steering Group on Clinical Leadership in the Ambulance Service (ACEG, 2009a)		

experience and expertise, and supported by the appropriate education and training. This identification and nurturing of "local" or in-house experts or succession planning, are key elements for an organisations in developing clinical leadership.

Clinical leadership self-assessment tool

The self-assessment tool shown in *Table 3.2* was developed for organisations to help them assess their success in developing clinical leaders, and is based on the four key elements of clinical leadership previously identified.

In 2007 the Department of Health commissioned a National Futures Leaders Study (NHS ACEG, 2009b) on behalf of ambulance services in England involving all 11 ambulance trusts. Twelve recommendations were made, each designed to support leadership development across middle to senior management with five recommendations directly related to clinical leadership:

- Recommendation 3 – to significantly strengthen the capacity for clinical leadership.
- Recommendation 4 – to actively participate in regional talent management initiatives.

- Recommendation 7 – to offer middle managers an accredited leadership programme, ideally with participants from other parts of the health system.
- Recommendation 8 – to develop clinical leadership through service improvement.
- Recommendation 11 – to develop the concept of a "productive ambulance team".

This study was important since it focused on the managerial aspect of clinical leadership and highlighted some current gaps in the service. Specifically the study pointed to significant capacity pressures in line management that resulted in clinical supervision being overlooked. Operational pressures to achieve national performance targets also contributed to the lack of clinical support and supervision of staff. The study concluded that it was necessary to establish a "culture of clinical professionalism" and to reinforce the shift from training to education (NHS Ambulance Chief Executive Group, 2009b).

Leadership versus management

At first glance the difference between leadership and management can appear vague. It is often quoted that "leaders do the right thing whilst managers do things right". While such quotations may or may not be true, leadership is just one of the many assets of a successful manager, although clearly care must be taken in distinguishing between the two concepts in practice. Managers will often do things "by the book" thus following organisational policy, while leaders follow their own intuition which may, in turn, be of more benefit to the organisation. Leaders tend to be more emotional than managers and when a natural leader emerges in a group already containing a manager, conflicts may arise if they have differing views. There is often greater loyalty to leaders rather than to managers and such loyalty is generated by the leader taking responsibility, for example, when things go wrong; by celebrating group achievements, even minor ones; and by giving credit where it is due. As such, leaders tend to be observant and sensitive people who know their team and develop mutual confidence within it.

Clinical leaders are individuals that others naturally follow through their own choice, whereas managers often hold a position of authority and therefore must be obeyed. Managers may only have obtained this authoritative position through time and loyalty to the organisation, not necessarily as a result of their managerial qualities. Managers are usually people who are experienced in their field and who have progressed through the organisation. Managers are well versed in the organisational hierarchy in which they work and may possess good technical knowledge. However, leaders may have little in the way of organisational skills, but their vision can unite teams. New leaders may have bold, fresh ideas but might not necessarily have experience or wisdom.

Therefore, management and leadership are two different ways of organising people. The manager utilises a formal, rational method whilst the leader uses passion and stirs emotions. It can be surmised that leaders tend to adopt the transformational model of leadership, whereas managers often adopt a more transactional approach.

Learning organisations

A learning organisation is one that should facilitate both individual and collective, or organisational, learning with a view to continuously changing itself and moving forward to new ways of working. The concept of a learning organisation suggests that learning and development is implicit within the organisation, not just a "bolt-on" or after-thought of the education and training policy. Key to this is the organisation's ability to adapt to change and to its external environment, to develop collective as well as individual learning and to utilise the results of learning to achieve better results (Department of Health, 2001a). The four key characteristics that a learning organisation has are:

- A *"learning culture"*. An organisation that nurtures a climate of learning.
- *Processes*. Those that encourage cross-boundary interaction such as infrastructure, development and management processes.
- *Tools and techniques*. Methods that aid individual and group learning, such as creativity and problem solving techniques.
- *Skills and motivation*. The ability to learn and adapt.

The most important point is that a learning organisation is not about more training. Training is obviously important in any organisation, but learning organisations will involve the development of higher levels of knowledge and skill.

With the rapid changes currently occurring within the NHS, the concept of organisational learning is more relevant today than ever to ensure the provision of high quality patient care. Organisational learning has been identified as a central concern for a modernised NHS and continuing professional development has an important role to play in improving learning of both the individual and the organisation (Davies et al, 2000). As such, the development of a learning organisation can provide benefits for the organisation, the individuals within it, and its customers or patients. The importance of both individual and organisational learning in the NHS was formally recognised in the *Working Together, Learning Together* document (Department of Health, 2001a), which sets out a strategy for lifelong learning in the NHS.

The value of applying knowledge, through collaborative working with other organisations such as primary care trusts and not just other directorates within ambulance trusts, for example, will improve patient care. Previously "collaborative working" was viewed as working with another directorate either within the organisation or with another ambulance trust. Working with other healthcare professionals will provide a different perspective of clinical care and the patient's journey. However, such collaboration is not always as systematic as it could be, but this potential should be harnessed to better match improvements in patient access to services and knowledge (Department of Health, 2001b). One example of good collaboration is that of ambulance services working collaboratively with intermediate care teams. Intermediate care teams provide short-term health and social care support and/or rehabilitation to patients in the community and consist of senior nurses, occupational therapists, physiotherapists and social workers amongst others. Intermediate care teams support early hospital discharge and admission avoidance programmes, assisting patients in the community with rehabilitation and facilitating independent living. Intermediate care teams also manage younger patients, who may have been discharged early, requiring treatment such as intravenous antibiotics for an infection. These patients may require cannulation, a skill that paramedic practitioners are able to teach the intermediate care team and also perform themselves as required.

In addition, the Social Care Institute for Excellence (2004) published a self-assessment resources pack that allows organisations to assess whether or not they are learning organisations.

Clinical leadership in practice

Applying clinical leadership to clinical practice from a paramedic, nursing or medical background has a number of similar core themes that will be discussed below. The rapid evolution of the paramedic profession has highlighted the importance of a solid organisational infrastructure for the success of clinical leadership. Evidence from recent ACEG documents (NHS ACEG 2009a, 2009b) offers an opportunity to observe the development and implementation of clinical leadership practice, and each professional group will be discussed.

Paramedic practice

The changing nature of the ambulance service in recent years, in conjunction with the additional demands of academic preparation and the developing professionalisation of the paramedic, has led to an increasing need for ambulance trusts to nurture and apply clinical leadership within their organisations, despite recognised organisational pressures.

The need for clinical leadership was also emphasised by David Nicholson, NHS Chief Executive, at the Clinical Leadership Summit in February 2007 when he suggested that clinical leadership worked best when:

- It was adopted at a local level, where it often effects the most change.
- Simple ideas are implemented by empowered individuals.
- There is an accompanying infrastructure to assist and support clinicians and managers in working together to ensure real changes to patient care.

The NHS Leadership Centre also suggested that those organisations that invested in their staff had a greater likelihood of being successful (Williams, 2005). At an Ambulance Leadership Forum in April 2007, ambulance leaders highlighted the requirement to invest in clinical leadership alongside other leadership and management developments, with a number of key themes emerging:

- The requirement to build clinical leadership capacity within the context of an overall paramedic career framework.
- Continuing clinical leadership from clinical to managerial roles.
- Clinical engagement from non-clinical managers and how these can best be linked.
- Clarity regarding the attributes of clinical leaders and how these can be supported through education and training.
- Supporting clinical leaders to play a larger role in service reforms beyond the response time targets.

Clinical leadership within ambulance services has traditionally been the primary responsibility of the medical director. These doctors frequently originated from trauma/acute care backgrounds, often working in isolation. As ambulance service delivery has changed over recent years fewer patients are being transferred to the emergency department with more patients being treated appropriately and managed at home. Consequently, the potential clinical risk has increased. The need for appropriately prepared leaders with experience and influence in such situations is crucial. For example, paramedics now manage a wider range of clinical scenarios than ever before.

The document *Taking Healthcare to the Patient* (Department of Health, 2005) proposed a number of radical changes to ambulance services in England, notably regarding clinical leadership. For example, Recommendation 62 stated:

There should be improved opportunity for career progression, with scope for ambulance professionals to become clinical leaders. While ambulance trusts will always need clinical direction from a variety of specialties, they should develop the potential of their own staff to influence clinical developments and improve and assure quality of care.

The NHS ambulance services could potentially develop patient and public involvement in clinical leadership programmes. Patients are keen to work with clinical leaders who understand their needs and aspirations and who can apply the insights and experiences of local people to develop effective and responsive urgent care programmes. For patients with long-term conditions and their carers, there is a role in customising the design and implementation of integrated NHS care, especially where transport services have a profound impact on longer-term well-being.

The *Future Role and Education of Paramedic Ambulance Service Personnel* (JRCALC/ASA, 2000) report proposed that both paramedic education and experience needs to be broadened and improved with a more coordinated approach to higher education.

The Allied Health Professionals Leadership Challenges Project involved allied health professionals in 10 Strategic Health Authorities across England. The aim of the project was to tap into the wealth of skills and expertise and use this experiential learning to develop and nurture innovative practice with the aim of improving patient care.

Nursing practice

Clinical leadership within nursing is better established. The RCN Clinical Leadership Programme (Royal College of Nursing, 2010) promotes achievement within the following specific areas:

- Policy influence and implementation.
- Strategic influence and function.
- Service improvement.
- Practice development.
- Personal development.

A recent report on the programme concluded that it was making a difference, with nurses gaining confidence and feeling empowered to lead their teams in spite of difficult circumstances (Large et al, 2005). Other key finding suggested that there was a strong link between stress, efficiency, performance and leadership. One programme participant stated: "If one was to select a 'strap line' to promote leadership, one could say that 'it gets to the bits that management can't reach'."

Similarly the Kings Fund Leadership Development Programme prepares individuals working at all levels in the health service to develop their leadership skills. Their approach is based on the knowledge, perceptions and assumptions that participants contribute in the problem-solving processes and the management of change.

Examples of clinical leadership roles in nursing include station managers or clinical supervisors, who provide clinical supervision and mentorship, supporting clinicians in both practice and education/training settings. These individuals also require further development for their own leadership skills, particularly to support

Setting direction
- Identify contexts for change – awareness of factors
- Applying knowledge and decisions – gathering evidence-based information
- Making informed decisions
- Evaluating impact

Personal qualities
- Self-awareness
- Self-management
- Self-direction – continuing professional development
- Acting with integrity (openly and ethically)

Working with others
- Working within teams
- Encouraging contribution
- Building and maintaining relationships – listening to and supporting others
- Developing networks – partnership working

Managing services
- Planning – actively contributing to service goals
- Managing resources – awareness and effective utilisation
- Managing people – providing direction and reviewing performance
- Managing performance – accountability

Improving service
- Ensuring patient safety – assessing and managing risk
- Critically evaluating – thinking analytically
- Encouraging innovation – continuous service improvement
- Facilitating transformation – contributing to change process

Figure 3.2. Medical leadership competency framework – delivering the service (adapted from NHS Institute for Innovation and Improvement, 2009).

newly qualified graduate nurses entering clinical practice. Research undertaken by Taylor (2008) suggested the need for "hybrid" roles – those that combine clinical practice and formal positions of leadership within an organisation. Such roles would facilitate the development of new skills whilst providing a direct route for knowledge and learning that can be incorporated into clinical practice.

Medical practice

From a medical perspective, the NHS Institute for Innovation and Improvement developed a Medical Leadership Competency Framework that aim to engage doctors in clinical leadership (see *Figure 3.2*). This Framework outlines five identified competencies to provide a tool to support involvement of planning, delivery and transformation of services and has been utilised in medicine for a number of years.

Although developed primarily for medical practitioners, this framework is based on the concept of shared leadership, where leadership is not restricted to a designated role and there is a sense of "shared responsibility". This potentially maps better with pre-hospital care delivery, as often medical and non-medical practitioners work in close alliance in this area. The overall competencies have been mapped to the previously identified elements of clinical leadership.

Implementing clinical leadership into practice

How clinical leadership is developed and implemented will vary between organisations; since one size does not fit all. The aim of the clinical leadership document (NHS ACEG, 2009a) was to develop a framework for practice that could be utilised by each organisation as required. A key element to ensure success was that whatever implementation model was adopted, clinical leadership is about clinical staff at all levels being actively engaged in the continuous improvement of the quality and safety of patient services – obviously easier said than done. It takes commitment and engagement from all directorates within an organisation – not just the clinical and/or organisational development directorates within a trust. Competing against the ever-present Category A call (for life-threatening injury/illness) response targets that need to be met amongst additional clinical governance issues, clinical leadership does not always feature highly on the agenda.

However, as a starting point, one of the key building blocks of leadership is a solid foundation in clinical practice. Clinical practitioners should develop relationships, whilst acting as role models, and encourage staff to listen to and support advocates who understand their values and challenges, thereby sustaining the improvements and changes introduced. The suggested components that constitute clinical leadership are based on the knowledge, skills and attributes outlined in *Table 3.1*.

The revised Paramedic Association Curriculum Guidance and Competence Framework (2008) outlines specific roles for the future ambulance clinician based on the Skills for Health Career Framework (see *Figure 1.1* in *Chapter 1*). Work undertaken by a national working group on clinical leadership in the ambulance service, proposed a clinical leadership ladder (NHS ACEG, 2009a).

Clinical leadership ladder

A clinical leadership ladder was developed by the National Steering Group to demonstrate the potential career progression of ambulance staff within

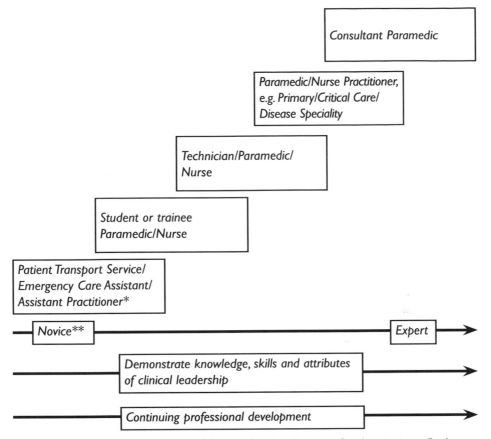

*Figure 3.3. The adapted clinical leadership ladder. See text for description of roles.
*Title may vary depending on trust; **Novice refers to an individual new to a role.*

an organisation. It was based on the Skills for Health Framework and therefore also maps the career development of other practitioners, such as nurses. Each level is relatively self-explanatory and describes the increasing level of responsibility and expertise required for each "step" of the ladder from the relative "novice" of an emergency care assistant to the consultant paramedic (see *Figure 3.3*). The ability to climb the ladder needs support with continuing professional development and ongoing commitment within the organisational structure.

The ladder can be "stepped off" at any time – individuals do not have to progress further up the ladder, but the opportunity should be made available for them to do so if they wish. Currently senior positions within ambulance trusts are limited and it should be recognised that, in reality, a limited number of individuals will succeed to the top "rung" but this has potential to increase in the future. Whilst the ladder was originally developed for use in the ambulance service, it could arguably be extrapolated to other urgent care professionals and the nursing profession. This is clearly not an exhaustive ladder – there are many potential adaptations and a variety of titles for the range of various practitioners, however some elements of this may be useful for application in other organisations and settings.

Some examples of the what the different roles involve are:

- *Patient Transport Service/Emergency Care Assistant/Assistant Practitioner*
  - Undertaking training programme
  - New to clinical practice
  - Recipient of preceptorship, mentorship
  - Supporting role to practitioners
- *Student or trainee Paramedic/Nurse*
  - IHCD or HEI/Diploma/FdSC/Dip
  - Works to established clinical standards/guidelines (JRCALC/MNC/QAA)
  - Beginning to use reflective practice
  - Self-regulation
- *Technician/Paramedic/Nurse*
  - HE Diploma/FdSc/Dip
  - Completed mentoring programme
  - Takes responsibility for others
  - Higher Education Mentorship module
  - Undertakes role of formal mentor/preceptor
  - Links to professional self-regulation (HPC)
  - Undertaking continuing professional development
  - Shared learning
- *Paramedic/Nurse Practitioner, e.g. Primary/Critical Care/Disease Speciality*
  - Educated to BSc
  - Undertaking specific academic programme at Masters level
  - Mentorship role
  - Reviews and develops policy and guidelines
  - Leads on clinical governance
  - Liaises with higher education institutions for academic quality
  - Acts as a resource to other practitioners
- *Advanced Paramedic/Senior Nurse Practitioner*
  - Educated to MSc
  - Lead clinical supervisor role
  - Reviews policy and guidelines
  - Takes a lead in organisational development
  - Expert resource for support/guidance
  - Participates in audit and research
  - Participates and reviews Serious Untoward Incidents/Patient Safety Alerts

- Manages and investigate clinical complaints
- Liaises with other healthcare professionals/trusts/practitioners
- *Consultant Paramedic*
  - Minimum of Masters degree
  - Undertaking study at PhD level
  - Expert clinical resource
  - Organisational development role
  - Developing new areas of clinical practice
  - Strategic/Executive Board membership
  - Developing new care pathways
  - Liaising with central healthcare policymakers
  - Instigating and reviewing care pathways
  - Instigating/undertaking primary research
  - Publishing and presenting at conferences

Box 3.1 Examples from practice

Admission avoidance for chronic obstructive pulmonary disease (COPD) patients
- Identify need for new guidelines for admission avoidance for patients suffering with acute exacerbations of COPD
- Liaise with local respiratory physician, clinical nurse specialist and pharmacist to develop and implement new care pathways
- Establish pilot group to trial new pathways
- Provide additional education/training for patient assessment and history-taking

Education practice facilitators
- Identify existing clinical tutors to support graduate/academic students in practice as "professional buddies"
- Liaise with universities, tutors, clinical managers, station and operational managers
- Provide on-site support and teaching
- Facilitate mentorship and clinical supervision

Enhancing continuing professional development (CPD)
- Develop and disseminate a standard CPD portfolio template
- Organise and deliver CPD workshops across the organisation to demonstrate CPD activities
- Set up local groups to run ongoing CPD sessions
- Ensure delivery of ongoing CPD, e.g. journal articles, DVDs, conferences, etc.

Box 3.1 cont/

---

e-learning
- Identify a small team of individuals to develop an e-learning strategy
- Liaise with Information Management and Technology team to develop a functional, accessible website – linked to Moodle, NHS Core Learning Unit (CLU)
- Pilot small teams to test CLU non-clinical mandatory training
- Disseminate information electronically, e.g. DVDs, thumb drives, CDs etc.

Leadership and management development
- Accessing the Exploring Leadership and Self-Awareness Programmes for middle managers
- Accessing similar programmes for senior managers
- Accessing Institute of Leadership and Management for team leaders
- Coaching development for black and minority ethnic staff

Working in practice

The report of the National Steering Group on Clinical Leadership in the Ambulance Service was intended to be a framework for practice. There are practical examples from practice that may be relevant to other organisations shown in *Box 3.1*. These are aimed at providing some practical ideas that might be useful and appropriate for local implementation.

To achieve successful implementation of clinical leadership, the evidence to date suggests that some of the basic skills needed include:

- Managing change
- Communication
- Negotiation
- How to engage staff
- Involvement with commissioning.

There are some key questions to consider prior to beginning with any clinical leadership activity. *Table 3.3* outlines a list of prompt questions that clinicians should consider prior to commencing any clinical leadership activity.

Table 3.3. What to ask before commencing with clinical leadership

Question	Purpose	Method
What will it look like?	To identify the structure of clinical leadership	Ensue that when clinical leadership activities are set up, thought is given to its structure and relationship to the bigger organisation.

Will it last?	To ensure sustainability	Small pilot projects are a good method to assess the potential impact of a larger activity within an organisation. Sustainability is frequently overlooked, resulting in failure and disillusionment of individuals. In order for any clinical leadership activity to be successful, sustainability from the wider organisation is vital
How big will it be?	To ascertain size of project	Small steps are often more successful than giant leaps. Developing the role of the front line clinical supervisor or leader, for example, may have a much more effective impact than introducing a senior, top-down role onto the organisation
Will it grow on me?	To nurture current expertise	Many individuals are keen to develop their professional role given the right support and guidance. Previously unrecognised talent or expertise that otherwise would have gone unnoticed or underutilised, can often be better advanced by providing additional education and training from within the organisation. Rather than importing, better to "grow your own" when it comes to developing aspects of specialist practice
Will it fail?	To address good succession planning	The lack of developing and/or implementing effective succession planning often relates to failure in developing clinical leadership. Much greater thought and preparation, linked to organisational aims and development targets, need to be considered in relation to developing individuals
How much time will it take?	To ensure protected time for activities and preparation	Releasing individuals from their operational/ managerial duties for professional and personal development is always challenging, particularly in the urgent care setting, where the priority is the clinical need of patients. Despite much discussion about the need for development, the lack of protected time and funding for release for individual development can become detrimental to the whole organisation

Who do I need to talk to?	To ensure collaboration between managers and leaders	Management and leadership activities are not necessarily mutually exclusive – an individual can be both a leader and manager. However the roles are significantly different and therefore care needs to be taken if the assumption is that all managers are leaders. This is often not the case and a good manager may not necessarily make a good leader and vice versa. This relates back to the previous point of a good clinical leader not necessarily being in a senior or "top" position

Best practice flowchart

A best practice flowchart was also developed as part of the report of the National Steering Group on Clinical Leadership in the Ambulance Service to assist practitioners to become clinical leaders (NHS ACEG, 2009a). The flowchart summarises the suggested stages in developing and implementing clinical leadership within an organisation. The steps are consecutive, although can be accessed at any point, depending on the organisation and based on the elements of clinical leadership, personal mastery, enabling team learning, developing a shared vision and systems thinking (see *Figure 3.4*)

Yorkshire Ambulance Services' model

Yorkshire Ambulance Service has developed a model of clinical leadership where a clinical hub, staffed 24 hours a day by paramedics and emergency medical technicians in the 999 communications centres, provide clinical advice and access to response staff and the public. Emergency care practitioners provide further clinical and task expertise.

The introduction of paramedic practitioners and the recruitment of additional emergency care practitioners in the Yorkshire Ambulance Service add to the clinical expertise available to support the management of patients at home when they have an urgent, but not an emergency, need. This helps to prevent unnecessary transfer to emergency departments and allows patients' needs to be managed via appropriate clinical pathways into community services and primary care.

Clinical managers oversee clinical performance within each operational area. This is achieved through clinical team educators who support clinical staff in a ratio of 1:12 and provide the link into education and training. Their role is designed to provide work-based support, acting as mentors and providing clinical supervision to all operational staff, giving them assurance that the appropriate level of care is being delivered to patients.

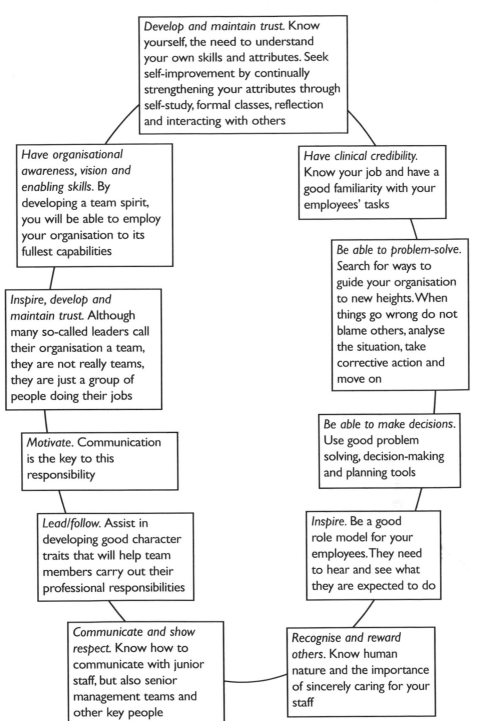

Figure 3.4. Best practice flowchart.

The educational needs of the clinical team educators and the ongoing development of the scheme are supported by the human resource and organisational development team.

The clinical directorate, consisting of the medical director, two assistant medical directors and an assistant clinical director with a nurse and paramedic background, provides clinical leadership. Clinical pathways advisors from both nursing and paramedic backgrounds support the pathway's links into primary and secondary care, as well as the regional clinical networks. The clinical excellence managers support clinical development and lead on clinical audit and clinical excellence.

The medical director leads dedicated clinical leadership days that involve a cross-section of staff in the organisation getting together to discuss clinical care, professionalism and leadership and to date over 100 members of staff have participated in these forums. This initiative is now involving staff from access and response teams so that clinical care is integrated into the initial point of contact for patients requiring assistance.

Conclusion

Clinical leadership transcends all directorates and is at the heart of developing and leading an organisation that delivers quality care. Clinical leadership relates to clinical governance, workforce planning, organisational development, education and training and continuing professional development to name but a few. Clinical leaders are positioned at all levels within the NHS and have a passion for their role, a clear picture of what they want their organisation to achieve, a special ability to share that vision with others and a talent for motivating, valuing and encouraging those around them (Mason, 2006).

References

Bass B, Avolio B (1990) *Transformational leading ability development. Manual for the Multifactor Leading Ability Questionnaire*. CA, USA: Consulting California Press

Benner P (2001) *From novice to expert: Excellence and power in clinical nursing practice* (Commemorative Edn). London, Sydney: Prentice Hall

Burns JM (1978) *Leadership*. New York: Harper & Row

College of Paramedics/British Paramedic Association (2008) *Paramedic Curriculum Guidance and Competence Framework*. Derbyshire: CoP/BPA

Cook MJ (2001) The renaissance of clinical leadership. *International Council of Nurses* 48(1): 38–46

Cook MJ, Leathard HL (2004) Learning for clinical leadership. *Journal of Nursing Management* **12**(6): 436–44.

Davies H, Nutley S, Mannion R (2000) Organizational culture and health care quality. *Quality Health Care* **9**: 111–19

Dawson S, Garside P, Hudson R, Bicknell C (2009) *The design and establishment of the Leadership Council*. Cambridge: University of Cambridge

Department of Health (1999) *Making a Difference – the nursing, midwifery and health visiting contribution. The midwifery action plan*. London: HMSO

Department of Health (2000) *The NHS Plan: A plan for investment, a plan for reform*. London: HMSO.

Department of Health (2001a) *Working together, learning together*. London: HMSO

Department of Health (2001b) *Shifting the balance of power: Securing delivery – Human resources framework*. London. HMSO.

Department of Health (2002) *Shifting the balance of power: The next steps*. London: HMSO

Department of Health (2004) *Overview of the NHS KSF*. London: HMSO

Department of Health (2005) *Taking healthcare to the patient: Transforming NHS Ambulance Services*. London: HMSO

Department of Health (2008) *Operating framework for the NHS in England 2009/10*. London: HMSO

Dreyfus H, Dreyfus S (2000) *Mind over machine. The power of human intuition and expertise in the era of the computer*. New York: Free Press

Gopee N (2008) *Mentoring and supervision in healthcare*. London. Sage

Health Professions Council (2007) *Standards of proficiency - Paramedics*. London: HPC

Johns (2003) Clinical supervision as a model for clinical leadership. *Journal of Nursing Management* **11**(1): 25–35

Joint Royal Colleges Ambulance Liaison Committee (2006) *UK ambulance service clinical practice guidelines*. Warwick: JRCALC

Large S, Macleod A, Cunningham G, Kitson A (2005) *A multiple-case study evaluation of the RCN Clinical Leadership Programme in England. Final report to the Royal College of Nursing and the NHS Leadership Centre, England*. London: RCN

Mason C (2006) What makes a good leader? *Primary Health Care* 16(10): 18–20

NHS Ambulance Chief Executive Group (ACEG) (2009a) *Report of the National Steering Group on Clinical Leadership in the Ambulance*

Service. London: ACEG

NHS Ambulance Chief Executive Group (ACEG) (2009b) *Future leaders study: The leadership capabilities and capacities of Ambulance Trusts in England*. London: ACEG

NHS Institute for Innovation and Improvement (2006) *NHS Leadership Qualities Framework*. Coventry: NHS Institute

NHS Institute for Innovation and Improvement (2008) *Medical leadership competency framework*. Coventry: NHS Institute

Nursing and Midwifery Council (2008) *Standards of conduct, performance and ethics*. London: NMC

Pintar KA, Capuano TA, Rosser GD (2007) Developing clinical leadership capability. *Journal of Continuing Education in Nursing* 38(3): 115–21

Quality Assurance Agency (2001) *Benchmark statement: Health care programmes Phase 1. Nursing*. Gloucester: QAA

Quality Assurance Agency (2004) *Benchmark statement: Health care programmes Phase 2. Paramedic science*. Gloucester:QAA

Quality Assurance Agency for Higher Education (2006) *Code of practice for the assurance of academic quality and standards in higher education. Section 6: Assessment of students*. Gloucester: QAA

Royal College of Nursing (2010) *Clinical leadership programme*. London: RCN

Schön DA (1983) *The reflective practitioner*. New York USA: Basic Books Inc

Social Care Institute for Excellence (2004) *Learning organisations: A self-assessment resource pack*. London: SCIE. Available from: http://www.scie.org.uk/publications/learningorgs/index.asp

Taylor J (2008) *Clinical leadership is central to the transformation of ambulance services. Engaging ambulance clinicians as leaders within their organisation will be a catalyst for change*. Unpublished dissertation. MSc Health Care Management, University of Birmingham

Timpson J (1998) The NHS as a learning organisation: Aspirations beyond the rainbow? *Journal of Nursing Management* 6(5): 261–74

Williams S (2005) *Literature review: Evidence of the contribution of leadership development for professional groups makes in driving organisations forward*. A Summary of a Report for the NHS Leadership Centre. Oxfordshire, England

CHAPTER 4

Clinical supervision

Clinical supervision has a number of interpretations, with many of the traditional models being more closely associated with nursing and allied health professions. Within the paramedic profession, clinical supervision is often not closely aligned to any identifiable model and practitioners are not provided with the protected time required in which to develop and implement this professional support.

It generally takes time to establish clinical supervision and to embed it into professional practice. It can be challenging to introduce it into a profession that has not previously either experienced effective clinical supervision or where poor supervision was offered. This chapter offers a description and overview of the key elements required to be an effective clinical supervisor, with some suggested models for urgent care and examples from practice. The term supervisee is used to identify the recipient of clinical supervision; supervisees can be either students or, more commonly in advanced practice, qualified staff that are developing their roles and practice.

Clinical supervisors in the NHS frequently have a dual role as supervisor and clinician, and therefore need to develop their coping skills for this dual role. A large amount of literature exists on the various clinical supervision frameworks and models available (Proctor, 1986, Heron, 1990, Sloan and Watson, 2001; Kavanagh et al, 2002). Many supervisors "learn on the job", and finding which model works best can depend on the supervisees, so it is important to encourage feedback to improve supervision and facilitate the learning process.

It is possible to distinguish clinical supervision from other more informal support mechanisms through the use of a contract. A contract establishes ground rules on issues such as confidentiality, commitment to attend, contribution to the session and the format of the supervision. Clinical supervision is not just about dealing with critical incidents or clinical or untoward errors but should be an ongoing accepted part of clinical practice. It should be a routine, implicit aspect for all clinical practitioners and it is arguably even more important in the advanced practice of urgent care.

What is clinical supervision?

Kavanagh et al (2002) suggested that definitions of clinical supervision differ across groups or settings, but in general there were three elements important for it to be effective. These are:

1. Improvement of clinical practice, e.g. problem-solving, learning new skills.
2. Professional support.
3. Quality assurance.

Perhaps the most important of these elements is that clinical supervision is a method by which to improve clinical practice. As such, one of the most appropriate definitions for clinical supervision is:

> *... a working alliance between practitioners in which they aim to enhance clinical practice ... meet ethical, professional and best-practice standards ... while providing personal support and encouragement in relation to professional practice.*
>
> (Kavanagh et al, 2002: 247)

Gopee (2008) defined clinical supervision as a peer-support role that was based in the clinically focused professional relationship between the practitioner and clinical supervisor. Having undergone some form of educational or academic preparation for the role, clinical supervisors could utilise their clinical knowledge and experience to assist supervisees/students to develop their own knowledge, competence, values and practices.

Evidence suggests that certain characteristics within organisations are key to successful clinical supervision:

- Links to a national approach that views supervision as an element of clinical governance.
- Is supported by an implementation plan.
- Is led at organisational and team level.
- Has protected time for implementation and identification of "champions" at each level.
- Adopts a philosophy of clinical supervision, i.e. a common definition and framework.
- Has evidence of positive outcomes.
- Links clinical supervision to a system of appraisal and continuing professional development.

Approaches to clinical supervision

The most common approach to clinical supervision is that of one-to-one supervision where a clinical supervisor supervises one individual – an approach that is popular in nursing (Girouard and Marchewka, 1983). A triad approach where a clinical supervisor supports two practitioners is also popular and group clinical supervision sessions offer a more time-efficient and collective approach that can be useful in problem solving (Sloan et al, 2000). Group supervision usually involves four to six practitioners being supervised by a sole supervisor. The kind of approach used is often dependent on staff release, clinical locations and the availability of an appropriate supervisor.

Clinical supervision models

Clinical supervision can be delivered in a variety of formats using a number of different models. Three models of clinical supervision will be discussed in this chapter although there are number of others models available and these are listed in the Resources section at the end of this chapter. The three models most suited to urgent care are:

1. Proctor's Three-Function Model (Proctor, 1986).
2. Heron's Six Category Intervention Analysis Framework (Heron, 1990).
3. The 4S Model.

Proctor's model

Proctor's model is commonly utilised in nursing due to its potential for diverse application. It is derived from counselling and has three "tasks" or functions (Proctor, 1986): the formative task, normative task and restorative task. During clinical supervision, the supervisor can focus on one or all three of the tasks at the same time, depending on the supervisee. The tasks are outlined further in *Table 4.1*.

The formative task is focused on learning and how to achieve the most from the session as a supervisee. This usually draws on the supervisees' experiential learning, often using a structured reflective framework in order to develop further knowledge and expertise. The focus of the normative task is accountability, encouraging supervisees to understand their roles and responsibilities and to clarify their boundaries in clinical practice. The restorative task is supportive and encourages staff to establish a support network and to undertake reflective practice in order to manage any issues arising from practice.

Proctor's model is not prescriptive and this can initially appear unhelpful. However the model should be viewed as a framework that allows supervisors to apply the tasks as required rather than feel that the model should dictate practice (Sloan and Watson, 2001). Although criticised by some (Brwkczynska, 1993), a study by Butterworth et al (1999) evaluating the effects of this model in nursing practice found it useful, demonstrating that working in the community or pre-hospital setting was more stressful than working in the hospital setting. This was compensated for by higher levels of job satisfaction and less emotional "burnout" in the pre-hospital setting.

91

Table 4.1. Proctor's Model of Clinical Supervision		
Action	Focus	Examples
Formative task		
Both supervisor and supervisee carry some degree of responsibility for the development of the students	Concerned with skills development and increasing supervisee's knowledge *Focus on learning*	Ensuring supervisee gets most from the session Explaining clinical supervision to others Using a structured reflective framework to aid reflection on practice Using experiential learning to develop further clinical knowledge and increase awareness of patient/client needs
Normative task		
Each carries a share of responsibility for ensuring that the student is adequately refreshed	Focuses on managerial issues including maintenance of professional standards *Focus on accountability*	Establishing roles and responsibilities in practice Clarifying of role boundaries in practice Addressing leadership potential Examining supervisee's role within the practice setting
Restorative task		
Both share a responsibility for the ongoing monitoring and evaluating of the students and either may carry the responsibility for assessment	Provides support to alleviate stress evoked by the job *Focus on support*	Managing own feelings from everyday workload Identifying and managing stress Recognising and establishing a support network Ensuring protected time for reflective practice and continuing professional development

With respect to the relationship between the nursing grade and stress, the higher the grade (i.e. the more experienced the nurse) the larger the workload, which is itself more stressful, whilst lower grade nurses found dealing with patients/relatives and balancing home and work life more stressful. Butterworth's study also demonstrated that whilst occupational stress levels were increasing, the rate of occupational burnout was not increasing. A key finding from the study was that stress management in nursing needs to be individually tailored, as not all nurses manage stress in the same way. This supported the model's flexibility – it can be adapted and used to meet the needs of individual groups.

Heron's Six Category Intervention Analysis Framework

Heron's six-category intervention framework analysis model has been adopted for clinical supervision and has two distinct aspects:

- A conceptual framework for understanding interpersonal relationships.
- A method for analysing a range of potentially therapeutic interactions between supervisor and supervisee.

Heron defined an intervention as being an identifiable piece of verbal and/or non-verbal behaviour that contributes part of the practitioner's service to the supervisee (Heron, 1990). In this model the emphasis is on what the practitioner intended to achieve in the intervention, rather than on the actual effect. The interaction is the practitioner taking on the role of listening to the "client" (or supervisee in this context) and the supervisee taking on the talking role.

Within Heron's framework there are two types of intervention; authoritative and facilitative, each of which is divided into three categories:

- Authoritative:
  - Prescriptive
  - Informative
  - Confronting
- Facilitative:
  - Cathartic
  - Catalytic
  - Supportive

In authoritative interventions, the supervisor takes a more dominant or assertive role, taking responsibility for and on behalf of the supervisee and this includes the prescriptive, informative and confronting categories. In facilitative interventions, the supervisor seeks to enable supervisees to become more autonomous and take more responsibility for themselves and includes the cathartic, catalytic and supportive categories. The categories are outlined further in *Table 4.2* which presents negative approaches that can be adopted by poor clinical supervision and which, of course, should be avoided. Some manipulative approaches include those where the supervisor is motivated by self-interest, often obvious when the supervisor insists on leading the session, not allowing the supervisee to lead (especially in the facilitative interventions). Similarly unskilled or incompetent supervision can occur as a result of lack of training or preparation of the supervisor who fails to grasp the realities of the situation. Studies suggest that Heron's framework is useful for the interpersonal aspect of the model and has been well-utilised in nurses' perceptions of their own interpersonal skills (Ashmore and Banks, 1997; Burnard and Morrison, 1988).

Table 4.2. Heron's Six Category Intervention Analysis Framework

Category	Negative approaches
Prescriptive	
Supervisor explicitly seeks to direct the behaviour of supervisee	Benevolent take-over. Creates dependency by giving advice to insecure supervisee who needs encouragement to be self-directing. Moralistic oppression. Encourages authoritarian approach by using "should", "ought" and "must" to supervisee who may appreciate this approach but feels impelled to reject the way in which it is presented.
Informative	
Supervisor seeks to impart knowledge, information and meaning to supervisee, by giving instruction	Seductive over-teach. Supervisor provides excessive information, so that supervisee becomes passive and moves away from self-directed learning. Oppressive over-teach. Supervisor is very verbal, provides too much information and is insensitive to the need of supervisee to contribute, preventing self-directed learning.
Confronting	
Supervisor seeks to raise supervisees' awareness of their behaviour and challenge any supervisee feedback	Sledgehammer. The supervisor raises issues aggressively, displacing their anxiety into an attack upon supervisees themselves rather than supervisees' attitudes or behaviour. The smiler. The supervisor says hurtful things to the supervisee in a smiling or jocular manner and any feedback is indirect and often confusing for supervisee.
Cathartic	
Supervisor assists supervisee to manage emotions, e.g. anxiety and anger	Encouraging dramatisation. Supervisor colludes with a supervisee to "act out" in destructive and disruptive ways. Nut cracking (too deep too soon). Supervisor makes too much of supervisee's distress, making supervisee defensive.
Catalytic	
Supervisor enables supervisee to learn, develop and problem-solve, encourages self-reflection and self-direction	Implicit take-over (compulsive search for order). Supervisor unwarily imposes some meaning into supervisee's experience – this intervention centres on the supervisor's, not the supervisee's search for learning. Scraping the bowl. Supervisor goes beyond the point of productive discussion, trying to enable the supervisee to find more to talk about in one area.
Supportive	
Supervisor seeks to clarify supervisee's attitudes, beliefs and actions	Moral patronage (or your character is coming along nicely). Supervisor loudly and publically praises supervisee, resulting in supervisee feeling insulted or "put down". Qualified support. Supervisor can only provide support to supervisee if the former discreetly reminds supervisee of some inadequacy.

The 4S Model

The 4S Model was developed by 16 NHS trusts in the Greater Manchester area as a model of clinical supervision for nurses and other allied health professionals (Waskett, 2009). The model was specifically developed for practitioners who were receiving clinical supervision for the first time that required a problem-solving approach. It was designed to be suitable for any healthcare professional. The result was a model that consisted of the following four stages:

Stage One: Structure

It is essential that the structure of the proposed supervision programme is established and senior members of the organisation are supportive of it to ensure that protected time is organised and agreed. The manager and team leader also need to agree on a structure in order to establish a clear framework for clinical supervision, and agree a policy. A number of issues need to be considered such as:

- *Should clinical supervision be optional or mandatory?* Optional is generally a better solution initially, since a mandatory requirement could overload the system and an optional approach allows time for raising awareness of the scheme.
- *Group or one-to-one sessions?* Group and single sessions offer different approaches and the choice may depend on the seniority of the staff and availability of the supervisor.
- *Timing of sessions?* One hour sessions on a monthly basis appear preferable for small groups.
- *Multidisciplinary?* There are advantages to working across disciplines, including awareness of other professionals, avoiding just using close friends and utilising supervisors from other professions (superior clinical knowledge is not usually necessary for clinical supervision).
- *Available resources?* Dependent on workloads, staff release and room availability. It is better to offer specific sessions and to keep to them rather than offer whole range of sessions.
- *Evaluation?* Consideration of how the outcomes will be measured and evaluated. It is worth having a discussion with the audit group?
- *Developing contracts and protocols.* Sharing template contracts and protocols/policies from other organisations and trusts may be useful.
- *Logistics?* Supervision works best when the supervisee(s) select the supervisor. It is perhaps worth speaking to other organisations regarding their experience, having a small selection of potential supervisors and considering looking outside the NHS.

Stage Two: Skills

Clinical supervisors should be adequately prepared for their role and there is a range of clinical supervision programmes available, e.g. in-house programmes, academic higher education institution modules and commercially available programmes. A solution-focused approach is often useful in healthcare since this is easily understood by practitioners, although it can be challenging as clinical staff are used to problem-solving but often not solution-building, which can take time to understand. It is also worth remembering that clinical supervisors do not necessarily need to be highly knowledgeable in the subject area of their supervisees. In fact it is often preferred that supervisors are from another discipline, facilitating greater objectiveness on the part of the supervisor.

Stage Three: Support

Providing support for clinical supervision is essential, and ensuring "sign up" by the organisation at the beginning of the process is vital. Clinical supervisors play a very important role in providing objective and positive support for their supervisee(s) and it is important that the supervisors themselves receive support. Peer support from colleagues is valuable and supervisors should meet regularly as a group. It can become an easy option to engage or revert to a didactic teaching session, moving away from the central ethos of support.

Stage Four: Sustainability

Sustainability is perhaps one of the biggest challenges in any new practice introduced into healthcare, particularly in urgent care where the achievement of a number of national targets, and the very unpredictable nature of the service often makes sustainability challenging. All too frequently the knee jerk response, when an organisation fails to meet national response targets, is the cancellation of all "non-urgent" activities, such as mentor meetings, continuing professional development activities and, potentially, supervision.

Waskett (2009) outlined some fundamental ways to encourage sustainability. These included:

- Ring fencing of financial resources.
- Identifying an overall leader who monitors, manages and evaluates the process.
- Facilitating supervisors to have access to relevant programmes and courses.
- Ensuring that new staff are incorporated into clinical supervision and that it is mapped to the NHS Knowledge and Skills Framework and is an element of appraisal.
- Regular reviewing and updating of policy documents.
- Evaluating clinical supervision.
- Ensuring that the clinical supervision model is suitable for the local situation.

Quality assurance and clinical supervision

Clinical supervision can be perhaps best summarised as clinical "super"-vision where practitioners have "super" vision to be able to view and guide fellow practitioners in their practice. Whichever clinical supervision model is adopted, it should be reviewed and evaluated regularly. Ask and Roche (2005) suggested that quality clinical supervision should increase supervisees' ability to reflect on and analyse critically their clinical practice. They also suggested that occasional observation by the supervisor of the supervisee's practice may also be helpful.

The supervisee's knowledge of evidence-based "best practice" in their specific field and their understanding of theoretical perspectives should also be developed, although teaching is not an element of the supervisor's role since they are focused in supporting the healthcare professional. Supervision should also identify and define areas for further professional development. Ask and Roche (2005) also suggested that to ensure continued high quality of supervision, clinical supervisors must be:

- Open and trusting.
- Non-judgemental.
- Affable.
- Highly accessible.
- Up-to-date in their knowledge of evidence-based interventions.
- Have the ability to impart skills.

Elements of successful supervision

Ideally for clinical supervision to be successful clinical supervisors need to be educated in the process of supervision. This includes aspects such as the contractual agreement between supervisor and supervisee, the frequency and timing of meetings, confidentiality issues and content, e.g. the clinical issues and competencies that need to be addressed.

The contractual agreement

Supervisees should be clear regarding the purpose and structure of the clinical supervision and this can be clearly defined in the clinical supervision contract. This contract should be drafted and discussed in the first session between the supervisee(s) and supervisor. Any specific aims, learning outcomes and objectives should be negotiated and monitored over an agreed time period. Clinical supervision should be conducted by principles of adult-centred learning, whereby supervisees determine the aims, objectives and the pace at which their learning occurs. This concept of "self-directed learning" is often relatively new to paramedics since their learning experiences to date have generally been through the traditional, didactic training approach. Nurses, in contrast, may be more familiar with self-directed learning and will be more comfortable with this approach.

Any identified learning that needs to be addressed should be agreed at the beginning of this process. For example, it may be the supervisee's first placement as a qualified paramedic. The supervisee's needs will vary in relation to any academic work or specific clinical targets and should be relevant and within salient clinical contexts. Learning specific clinical skills via observation can be a feature of supervision although the supervisor needs to ensure that they are not replicating any other teaching and assessment role available to the supervisee from individuals such as practice educators, tutors or mentors since this is not the usually an aspect of the clinical supervisor's role.

In general, clinical supervision sessions are for reflective discussion and analysis rather than teaching and/or assessment. The mode of contact should also be agreed. When one-to-one supervision is not possible in person then other methods of contact can be considered, such as email, telephone or use of video-conferencing, which can be very effective if there is geographical distance between supervisor and supervisee(s).

It is common for practitioners to be hesitant about clinical supervision since there are often popular misconceptions that supervisees' clinical practice and competency might be scrutinised or challenged or perhaps that line managers are "checking up" on their practice. Such misconceptions should be dispelled early in the process and significant amounts of time and energy may be required in order to ensure that supervisees have a clear understanding of the role of supervision. This also strengthens the argument for not using line managers as clinical supervisors. A sample contractual agreement for clinical supervision is outlined in *Figure 4.1*, although other local examples may be available.

Timing and scheduling of supervision

Edwards et al's (2005) study established that clinical supervision was more positively evaluated when monthly sessions lasted at least one hour. Other positive influences included supervision sessions that were conducted away from the clinical workplace and where supervisees selected their supervisor. While this study acknowledged that releasing staff for an hour on a monthly basis might be challenging, particularly in the urgent care setting such as the ambulance service, less frequent sessions appeared to be of limited value to the supervisee.

The allocation of adequate time for each supervision session also needs to be agreed and, as far as possible, adhered to. The usual timing for an average supervision session is one hour – as identified earlier, anything less is usually insufficient. It is difficult to specify the optimum frequency of supervision

Supervisee's contact details:			
Supervisor's contact details:			
Date of agreement:	Review date:		
Frequency of sessions:	Duration of session:	Venue of session:	
Supervisee's expectations			Achieved
• Anticipate support in clinical and professional practice			
• Review and support higher education institution's learning outcomes			
• Establish and monitor completion of clinical competencies			
• Develop reflective practice approach			
Supervisor's expectations:			Achieved
• Commitment to attend session. Inform promptly if unable to attend			
• Supervisee responsible for achievement of learning outcomes			
• Supervisee to maintain own documentation			
• Feedback to supervisee as necessary			
Maintain confidentiality			
• No disclosure of patient-identifiable information • No discussion of the session outside the supervisory session • Every individual is accountable for confidentiality • Any notes taken are private and confidential and remain the property of the supervisee			

Figure 4.1. Suggested clinical supervision contractual agreement (adapted from Macmillan, 2004).

sessions, since experienced or advanced practitioners generally require fewer sessions than less experienced or undergraduate staff. Frequency of sessions should be flexible and adapted as the role dictates and should be outlined in the contract. A student or less experienced practitioner may require a session fortnightly and may have a greater need for one-to-one sessions, whereas more experienced, advanced practitioners benefit from group sessions.

Ensuring protected time is made available is often extremely challenging. This is enormously frustrating for both supervisor and supervisee.

A clear distinction should be made between clinical supervision and line management/supervision as the two roles can be easily confused. Clinical supervision is focused on developing the practitioner's clinical roles and performance whereas line management/supervision is concerned with the evaluation and appraisal of all aspects of a practitioner's performance. It can be advantageous, although admittedly not always practical, to select a clinical supervisor who is external to the organisation and therefore independent of any of the issues and processes concerned.

Confidentiality

One of the most important tenets of clinical supervision is that of confidentiality. Healthcare practitioners are generally excellent communicators and therefore have a very clear understanding of confidentiality issues and accountability to patients, as outlined in their codes of professional conduct. Clinical supervisors need to help their supervisees explore the issues of confidentiality and identify and utilise their own strengths in this issue. As part of the contractual agreement, the supervisee should be informed about the limits of confidentiality and the necessities of any obligatory reporting at the beginning of the supervisory period.

Professional boundaries

The concept of observing professional boundaries in clinical supervision is very important. Clinical supervision is not therapy; supervision sessions should never become a counselling session for the supervisee's personal issues. There will inevitably be issues that impact on a practitioner's clinical performance and these can be identified in the supervision session and discussed, with some suggested sources of further support that the supervisee can seek elsewhere. This is an adult-based approach to supervision and should be clearly outlined in the contractual agreement. Obviously there should be no development of friendship or relationship beyond that of the supervision sessions, and again this should be clearly stated in the contract and explained at the first session.

There may, of course, be occasions when the supervisee and supervisor do not get along and this can be for a number of reasons. It could be that a group of supervisees working in a specific clinical area require a female supervisor, for example in women's health, and as such an appointed male supervisor would not be appropriate. We are all human and occasionally a supervisee and supervisor simply do not get along and continuing such an arrangement would be detrimental to the supervisory process and it may be necessary for the agreement to cease and for other provisions to be made. This is an unlikely occurrence, and a good supervisor will recognise such situations and implement a strategy to ensure that the supervisee can access suitable alternative supervision. As far as possible any specific requirements for the supervisee should be met.

After a prolonged period of supervision, a new face and change of approach may be required, and, as part of the review process, it may be necessary to change the supervisor. This can be done as part of the evaluation of supervision and it should be acknowledged that a new clinical supervisor with a fresh approach could further the supervisee's professional development.

Conclusion

Waskett (2009) described clinical supervision as similar to the Cheshire cat in Lewis Carroll's *Alice in Wonderland* in that it smiles broadly from on high but then tends to fade in and out of view. This can sometimes represent some organisations' approach to supervision; while some use it regularly, others mean to but somewhere along the line the practice and impetus dwindle. The importance of having support from senior management and an individual to oversee clinical supervision will help to ensure that clinical supervision can be successfully implemented into practice.

References

Ashmore R, Banks D (1997) Student nurses' perceptions of their inter-personal skills: A reexamination of Burnard and Morrison's findings. *International Journal of Nursing Studies* **34**(5): 335–45

Ask A, Roche AM (2005) *Clinical supervision: A practical guide for the alcohol and other drugs field*. Flinders University Adelaide Australia: National Centre for Education and Training on Addiction (NCETA).

Brwkczynska G (1993) Nursing values: Nightmares and nonsense. In Jolley M, Brwkczynska G (Eds) *Nursing: Its agendas*. London: Edward Arnold

Burnard P, Morrison P (1988) Nurses' perceptions of their interpersonal skills: A descriptive study using Six Category Intervention Analysis. *Nurse Education Today* **8**: 266–72

Butterworth T, Carson J, Jeacock J, White E, Clements A (1999) Stress, coping, burnout and job satisfaction in British nurses: Findings from the clinical supervision evaluation project. *Stress Medicine* **15**(1): 27–33

Edwards D, Cooper L, Burnard P, Hanningan B, Adams J, Fothergill A, Coyle D (2005) Factors influencing the effectiveness of clinical supervision. *Journal of Psychiatric and Mental Health Nursing* **12**(4): 405–14

Girouard S, Marchewka A (1983) Individual clinical supervision: A strategy for professional growth. *Topics in Clinical Nursing* **5**(3): 63–70

Gopee N (2008) *Mentoring and supervision in healthcare*. London: Sage Publications

Heron J (1990) *Helping the client. A creative practical guide*. London, Newbury Park, California: Sage

Kavanagh DJ, Spence SH, Wilson J, Crow N (2002). Achieving effective supervision. *Drug and Alcohol Review* **21**(3): 247–52

Proctor B (1986) Supervision: A co-operative exercise in accountability. In Marken M, Payne M (Eds) *Enabling and ensuring*. Chicago: University of Chicago Press

Sloan G, Watson H (2001) John Heron's six-category intervention analysis: Toward understanding interpersonal relations and progressing the delivery of clinical supervision for mental health nursing in the United Kingdom. *Journal of Advanced Nursing* **36**(2): 206–14

Sloan G, White CA, Coit F (2000) Cognitive therapy supervision as a framework for clinical supervision in nursing: Using structure to guide discovery. *Journal of Advanced Nursing* **32**(3): 515–24

Waskett C (2009) An integrated approach to introducing and maintaining supervision: The 4S model. *Nursing Times* **105**(17): 24–6

Resources

NHS Gateway to leadership programme: http://www.nhsgatewaytoleadership.co.uk/

NHS Institute for Innovation and Improvement – Leadership Qualities Framework: http://www.nhsleadershipqualities.nhs.uk/

Academic Clinical Leadership programmes - University courses (this list is not exhaustive)

Coventry University: http://www.coventry.ac.uk/cu/external/content/1/c4/51/76/v1238064393/user/Advancing%20Practice_MSc_03-2009_P.pdf

University of Bedfordshire: http://www.beds.ac.uk/courses/bysubject/heacar/msc-leaheapra

University of Leeds: http://www.healthcare.leeds.ac.uk/study/CPD/PG/multi-professional/PGC-LMHSC-08/details.htm

University of Warwick – Institute of Clinical Leadership: http://www2.warwick.ac.uk/fac/med/icl

Keele University: http://www.keele.ac.uk/depts/hm/cml/

RCN – Clinical Leadership Programme: http://www.rcn.org.uk/development/practice/leadership

NHS Institute for Innovation and Improvement – Improvement leaders guide: http://www.institute.nhs.uk/building_capability/building_improvement_capability/improvement_leaders%27_guides%3a_introduction.html

Academic Journals (will require personal or institutional subscription for access)

Emergency Medicine Journal: http://emj.bmj.com/

Journal of Paramedic Practice: http://www.paramedicpractice.com

Emergency Nurse Journal: http://www.rcn.org.uk/development/communities/

rcn_forum_communities/emergency_care/reading_room/emergency_
nurse_journal

Clinical Supervision Model

*Clinical supervision skills for nurses and allied health professionals: the 4s
model*: http://www.northwestsolutions.co.uk/supervision-4s-res.php

CHAPTER 5

Mentorship

Mentorship is a key element for professional practice, underpinning both student development and support for qualified staff in their own clinical and professional practice. Mentorship was formally introduced into nursing in the 1980s having initially been pioneered by Darling (1984) in the US. In the UK the then English National Board stipulated that training institutions were to ensure that clinical placements were supported with an agreed mentorship programme – although no specific information or guidelines were provided regarding delivery (Loads et al, 2006). Gray and Smith (2000) noted that mentorship was adopted by nursing in the UK largely unchallenged and suggested that little quality research exists as to whether mentorship was either successful or appropriate. The nursing diploma programme, Project 2000, further highlighted the requirement of mentorship with the introduction of more educational programmes for nursing.

Mentors were generally viewed as sharing their clinical experiences, thereby enhancing their mentee's skills and so furthering their own education and learning. This shared relationship was important since the aim was not simply to ensure students mirrored the actions of the mentor but a more collaborative relationship was required, ensuring the growth of knowledge in a safe and stimulating environment.

The concept of mentorship has been a key element of healthcare practice, specifically in nursing, for a number of years. This chapter outlines some of the definitions of mentorship, the issue of competence and performance and the theory–practice gap that can exist.

Definitions of mentorship

There is a range of definitions for mentoring and mentorship and also for similarly titled roles that support practitioners in practice:

- *Mentor*: An experienced professional, nurturing and guiding the mentee whether a student or established professional.
- *Assessor*: An experienced professional, making judgements on another's ability to carry out procedures or interactions.
- *Clinical supervisor*: An exchange between practising professionals to enable the development of professional skills and knowledge
- *Preceptor*. A teacher or instructor.

In general, students and newly graduated staff usually require mentorship and the term mentee is used in this chapter to denote the recipients of mentoring.

The role of the mentor is different from that of the nurse educator, which has been the traditional model for support to new staff. The nurse, as educator, usually taught nursing skills in a relatively didactic manner but this was frequently distanced from clinical practice and therefore such educators were often deskilled. Darling (1984) stated that there were in fact three aspects to the mentor role, that of inspirer, investor and supporter. Inspirers were individuals that mentees often "looked up to" or admired and Darling referred to this as "attraction" based on the fact that there is such a requirement for a successful mentor–mentee relationship. Successful mentors also needed to be investors, since mentors often invested their own time and energy in order to support and assist the student's development – what Darling referred to as "action". Thirdly, mentors were also supporters, as students required a positive attitude from their mentor. Darling described this as the "affect" element.

As noted, there are many terms used in relation to the whole concept of supporting mentees in their learning, such as "mentor", "facilitator", "preceptor" and "supervisor". These terms are often used interchangeably. Hagerty (1986) referred to this as a "definition quagmire" and suggested that with such a lack of consensus on definition how can anyone agree on what is meant by mentorship. Similarly, Donovan (1990) suggested that this lack of definition is further confused by the overlap with other roles, such as supervision and preceptorship, referring back to Darling's three suggested roles of inspirer, investor and supporter.

Qualities of an effective mentor

We may have a personal view of what makes an effective mentor based on personal experience. Gray and Smith's (2000) literature review highlighted the qualities of an effective mentor by identifying the mentor's key attributes (see *Table 5.1*). Being mentored effectively has been found to greatly improve the learning experience; mentored learning was more organised and structured and mentees reported that they were not just "tagging along" with their clinical peers. Gray and Smith also reviewed a study that explored the views of diploma students. They found that initially the mentees felt that the mentor was exclusively "theirs" – although this opinion evolved as the mentees began to appreciate the multi-faceted roles of the mentor. The mentees' dependence on their mentors appeared to be inversely proportional to their knowledge acquisition. Mentees quickly took advantage of any learning opportunities and, as they became more skilled and staff expectations of them increased, so their reliance on the mentor decreased. It also seemed that a "good" mentor with a "good" placement was, perhaps rather sadly,

Table 5.1. Attributes of an effective mentor		
Effective mentor attributes	*Role model*	*Teaching abilities/skills*
Genuinely interested in the student Has confidence and trust in the student's abilities Approachable and friendly Patient and understanding Sense of humour Spends time with the student Gradually withdraws support	Professional Organised Caring Self-confident Enthusiastic	Good communicator Knowledgeable about the relevant course Has realistic expectations of the student Paces their teaching Gives regular feedback Involves students in activities
		Adapted from Gray and Smith (2000)

viewed as luck or a happy coincidence. The study provides a useful checklist of the attributes or qualities of an effective mentor. It also outlines what is expected of a mentor from the mentee's perspective which includes finding their mentors as senior, knowledgeable and acting as a role model, as outlined in *Table 5.1*.

The mentees in Gray and Smith's (2000) study also identified what constituted poor mentorship practice (fortunately rare). They reported that poor mentors:

- Broke promises.
- Lacked knowledge and expertise.
- Had poor teaching skills.
- Lacked structure to their teaching.
- Changed their minds.
- Were over-protective of the students, e.g. did not let them participate in skills, etc.
- Delegated unwanted clinical tasks to students.
- Often disliked their own role and were disliked by their peers.
- Were distant and unfriendly.
- Were unapproachable and intimidating to students.
- Had unrealistic expectations of students.

Preparation of mentors

There is a wide range of training and educational programmes available to prepare practitioners for their mentorship role, either delivered in-house by trusts, or by higher education institutions, and are often part of undergraduate and postgraduate programmes. Nurses and a growing number of paramedics have experienced formal training and education throughout their careers. The majority of pre-registration courses in the previous two decades have witnessed a transition in their approach to learning and development. Some post-registration courses have also been training-based, reinforcing a variety of clinical skills, usually on a compulsory basis.

Training is essentially about providing knowledge and skills that are focused on a specific endpoint – usually followed by some form of assessment. Training is very often didactic – a traditional classroom-based activity, that favours rote-type learning. This approach served an adequate purpose for a number of years, but most healthcare professionals are now familiar with a more adult, educational approach to their learning.

Education, on the other hand can be defined as imparting valuable information, which is passed on and learnt. The student usually cares about the actual learning involved and what is being learnt has a place in the coherent pattern of life and therefore has relevance to their clinical practice.

Whichever approach to study is undertaken, a key aspect for mentors to learn is the need to develop effective relationships, since communication and negotiation are key skills required for effective mentoring. A good relationship between mentor and mentee is essential and usually develops, like any relationship, over time. In essence, the key relationship attributes are that mentorship should:

- Act as a resource.
- Work in an "observe and engage" relationship, offering a safe environment to assess new knowledge and skill, with the aim of growth and development.
- Work in partnership.
- Develop trust and openness in communication.
- Establish a "role model" relationship.
- Provide ongoing evaluation and development.

Mentees also reported that mentors should be viewed as a "supporter, guide, assessor and supervisor" (Gray and Smith, 2000: 545).

The mentoring role often creates an additional workload for practitioners, since mentorship is often in addition to a range of other clinical responsibilities, educational commitments and managerial or other operational duties. It frequently attracts no additional financial remuneration and therefore mentors are clearly committed, motivated individuals to start with.

Communication

Communication is clearly a key attribute in the mentor–mentee relationship. Excellent communication skills and techniques are paramount and communication methods will vary depending on the situation. However it will probably include one, or a combination of the following:

- *Written*: Handwritten documents (such as practice portfolios, clinical workbooks or similar), word processed documents, email, text, fax, printed handouts, e.g. relevant journal articles.
- *Verbal*: One-to-one telephone conversations, telephone conferencing with groups of mentees; open and closed questioning; using silence to elicit responses.
- *Non-verbal*: Observing body language, eye contact, posture, seating arrangements, etc.

The ability to communicate effectively with mentees is a skill that mentors need to possess. Senior and experienced practitioners undertaking the mentorship role, such as paramedics and nurses, are often exceptional at communication since the core element of their role in urgent care is to observe and rapidly assess situations. The use of a range of communication skills can assist the mentor to maintain contact and develop the all-important professional relationship with their mentee(s) whilst combining their other roles of clinician and often manager or educator.

Access to mentors

Ensuring access to mentors when required is key for mentees, particularly if there is an issue in practice. A recent study suggested that the current system of mentorship in the NHS is in crisis, urgently requiring an "overhaul" (Lakasing and Francis, 2005: 40). Mentors are experienced and respected professionals, often experts in their fields. Whilst this is clearly ideal for the mentorship role, the pressures of a mentor's often unpredictable clinical workload, particularly in the urgent care setting, can result in little time to devote to mentees. Also there are often high mentee:mentor ratios, contrary to the one-to-one ideal. As such, the mapping of mentor and mentee rotas often becomes increasingly logistically difficult, leading to reduced time in the mentoring role.

For paramedics involved in mentoring there is a need to include down time between calls to reflect and discuss cases with mentees. However, there is frequently pressure to attend the next call, but even a 30-minute break can assist both mentor and mentee in consolidating learning, and communicating with control regarding this is essential for effective mentoring.

Both medical and nursing professions acknowledge the challenge of remaining clinically updated. As nurses move from clinical practice into education and teaching roles, there is the potential for them to become out-dated regarding current clinical practice, resulting in a potential "theory–practice gap". The teaching of key clinical skills and competencies can sometimes be better delivered by a practising professional, such as a mentor. The introduction of paramedic lecturer-practitioners can assist in reducing some of this potential frustration in relation to teaching and assessing skills in practice, but such roles are not common (Corlett, 2000). The role of the lecturer-practitioner is discussed later in this chapter.

Mentor preparation

In the early 1990s, the nursing literature reported the challenges that faced nurse mentors in facilitating and assessing learning in clinical practice (Lankshear, 1990; Girot, 1993). Competency rating scales were developed and used in the 1960s but these were frequently outdated and were neither evidence-based nor consistent. Initially many of the mentor-assessed practice-based skills were very task-orientated, such as cannula insertion, wound dressings and so on and relied heavily on "rote" learning. This arguably provided only a snapshot of competence at a moment in time, not allowing for flexibility in patient-centred care.

Traditionally, mentors have been largely relied upon to assess clinical skills and the decreasing availability of link lecturers and clinical tutors in some clinical areas has increased the workload on mentors. It is also apparent that mentors are also often not fully prepared for this increasingly important element of their role. Price (2006) argued that there were three areas of concern for mentor preparation (see *Table 5.2*):

- Lack of preparation and competency of mentors themselves. As such, practitioners frequently have little in the way of formal educational preparation for the role, perhaps learning the skills on the job from when they have been mentored themselves.
- Lack of understanding of the structure and/or purpose of assessment.
- Lack of understanding of how constructive learning can be achieved.

Table 5.2. Areas of concern for mentor preparation	
Area of concern	*Context*
Preparation and competency of mentors themselves	• Mentorship programmes too short – only addressing the principles of supervision and assessment • Mentors often have issues regarding educational terminology, particularly if they are novices to an educational approach

The structure or purpose of assessment	• Confusion over whether the assessment is of:
	  • learning or a report on progress
	  • a performance of achievement, which will presume that there are some clear parameters against which to measure achievement

Achieving constructive learning in the clinical area	• Ensuring that performance and competence are judged fairly in the best way possible • Acquiring the skills to teach mentees effectively

These are key areas that need addressing in preparing mentors. There can be a lack of understanding by senior managers of the value and benefits of mentoring and therefore a reluctance to release staff for preparation such as via further education, training and continuing professional development opportunities.

Competence and performance

It is worth exploring some definitions of competence and performance since both terms are used interchangeably in mentoring, which can cause confusion.

Competence

One of the difficulties in discussing the issue of competence is the apparent lack of a clear definition of this important concept. It is interesting, and perhaps worrying, that whilst much is spoken and written about the assessment of competence, there is little in the way of its clarification.

The Health Professions Council (HPC) has no clear definition for either the term "competence" or "competency". The Department of Health's *Allied Health Professions Project: Demonstrating competence through continuing professional development* defined competence as "the complex synthesis of knowledge, skills, values, behaviours and attributes that enable individual professionals to work safely, effectively and legally within their particular scope of practice" (Department of Health, 2003: 9).

In relation to professional practice and competence, the Quality Assurance Agency's (QAA) subject benchmark statements outline the expectations in a range of subject areas, including paramedic practice. Each benchmark statement identifies and defines what can be expected of graduates in terms of their "abilities and skills which illustrate understanding of and competence in the subject" (QAA, 2010: 7).

Although not directly related to paramedic practice, the Nursing and Midwifery Council (NMC) offer a loose definition of competence: "the skills and abilities to practise safely and effectively without the need for direct supervision" (NMC, 2008: 45).

Perhaps more closely related to paramedic practice, in pre-hospital medicine, Clements and Mackenzie (2005: 516) suggest "achievement of competence requires demonstration of a defined range of underpinning knowledge, psychomotor skills, and behavioural attributes".

These definitions focus on the acquisition of knowledge, skills and attributes that are the cornerstones in learning. As such, competence-based and assessed education programmes should clearly define the term competency to avoid unnecessary confusion. They should also outline the competences and

Table 5.3. Benner's Novice to Expert Model: developmental phases

Stage	Descriptor	Development phases	CoP/BPA Career Framework	
1. Novice	No experience of situation in which they are expected to perform – rule-governed behaviour	Moving from reliance of abstract principles to using prior experience to support actions	1–4	
2. Advanced beginner	Demonstrate marginally acceptable performance			
3. Competent	Clinician in same role for 2-3 years, able to cope and manage complex situations			
4. Proficient	Understand situation as a "whole" – perceptions based on prior experience	Viewing situations holistically and selecting relevant sections for action	5–6	
5. Expert	No longer relies on analytical principle – huge background of experience with an intuitive grasp of situations	Moving from detached observer to involved performer, becoming engaged in the situation	7–9	
CoP – College of Paramedics; BPA – British Paramedics Association				

their various subsets that are required to be achieved for successful completion of the programme of study. Paramedics and nurses would therefore have much greater clarity on the number and complexity of competences by which they are to be assessed.

Benner's (2001) Model of Skill Acquisition has its foundations in nursing and Benner identifies "competent" in Stage 3 in her Novice to Expert model. Benner's Model (as seen in *Table 5.3*), which is applicable to all healthcare professions, states that the competent nurse (or practitioner) is "typified by the nurse (or practitioner) who has been on the job in the same or similar situation for two or three years, develops his/her actions in terms of long-range goals or plans of which he/she is consciously aware (Benner, 2001: 25; Dreyfus and Dreyfus, 2000).

One could argue however that if a practitioner only achieves competence following two to three years in a role then are practitioners competent when they qualify and first register with their professional body? This is an interesting dilemma and one that merits further research. Reflecting on your own experience on initially qualifying as a paramedic or nurse, could you claim to be a "competent" practitioner at that stage, compared to today?

Performance

Similarly to competence, there is little consensus in the literature with regard to the definition of performance. Again While (1994) proposed that performance is suggestive of high quality care involving cognitive, affective and psychomotor skills. Factors that appear to influence a mentee's performance include the clinical placement, whether there are formal/informal codes of conduct, the type and variety of patients, and general placement morale. This morale relates to mentees' overall feelings of value and their ability to achieve a difficult task, which increases their self-value and self-esteem. One might recall a particularly enjoyable placement for a variety of reasons, and this feeling of enjoyment probably also had a beneficial impact on your performance.

Linking competence and performance

Linking competence and performance is key in mentoring students. "Hands on" manual skills were once thought to be the only useful assessment measure for healthcare students. For example, the ability to undertake a task such as preparing an infusion with a therapeutic additive would be observed and graded. Although an assessment of this common skill is valuable, it does not take into account higher-level decision-making skills, such as the ability to calculate the correct drug dosage to be added and the ability to ascertain if the additive was actually clinically required. These skills are as important as the manual skill of infusion preparation.

Black and Wolf (1990) suggested that competence should relate to the ability to perform effectively on different occasions (not just on one occasion) and in different contexts. The ability to achieve a "competence" on one specific day does not of course necessarily equate to mentees being "competent". This common dilemma often causes discomfort in clinical assessors who rightly feel uncomfortable in "signing off" a student to be competent when they have only witnessed a competence on one occasion. The reassurance is that by signing, timing and dating the competence, they are merely stating that the mentee was competent on that particular day and in that particular context. Competency assessment should, of course, be continuous and develop through the programme of study.

The advantages of such continuous assessment are that it facilitates the personal development of the mentee thereby "averaging" out the days when students perform less well, assisting the students in progressing towards their final learning objective/outcome and perhaps providing a better overall view of performance. The disadvantages of continuous assessment are that such close supervision in practice is time and resource intensive and not always practical, often requiring lengthy documentation (Hand, 2006).

The theory–practice gap

The theory–practice gap, literally the potential breach between the theoretical frameworks and clinical practice, can create barriers to effective learning. Corlett's (2000) literature review explored the theory–practice gap from the perspective of tutors, student nurses and clinical preceptors and discovered that whilst it did not appear that qualified staff lacked the appropriate knowledge, the application of theory to practical situations was difficult. However some tutors felt this "gap" was actually beneficial – encouraging students to develop problem-based learning and reflective skills. Perhaps not surprisingly, the students did not share this view, reportedly feeling frustrated by it (Corlett, 2000).

Many idealised views of practice are not always apparent in reality. For example, academic lecturers may teach a cannulation technique only for students to discover in clinical practice that the taught approach is now considered out of date. Exploring and understanding this local context can assist in understanding mentees' frustration, hence the role of the lecturer-practitioner is often popular with mentees and staff (see below for a description of the lecturer-practitioner role). Corlett (2000) referred to this problem as "idealism versus realism" and in fact it is often well managed by some mentees, who utilise their problem-solving skills to practise within their own parameters, although less mature or junior students could find this difficult to resolve.

Another contributing factor to the theory–practice gap is that mentors often have little time in which to develop effective relationships with their mentee(s). Corlett referred to "sequencing" or ensuring the relevant theory was taught immediately prior to a clinical placement. For example, students working on a rapid response vehicle or on a cardiac care unit caring for patients with acute chest pain would find the experience challenging without having been taught the educational theory relating to the cardiovascular system prior to the placement. Often the starting point for the mentoring relationship is the students themselves and their knowledge and learning to date.

Closing the theory–practice gap

Having identified a gap, understanding how best to close, or at least reduce, it is an important issue. Corlett's (2000) study identified three key areas for reducing the gap:

- Improved communication.
- Information sharing.
- Collaboration.

It is also possible that students only experience theoretical relevance retrospectively – often in an idealistic and decontextualised way as the relevance of theory to practice only becomes evident after some time spent consolidating their learning. Corlett (2000) argued that the theory–practice gap is a problem mentees have to bear until such time as they have sufficient knowledge and experiential understanding to fit the various aspects of theory and practice together for themselves. Not all learning can be taught in the classroom. Mentees are required to know the relevance of what they are being taught and have the ability to apply it; the "know that" and the "know how" of the different types of knowledge, with the former being gained from theory and education and the latter from experience in the clinical setting (Benner, 2001).

Teaching tutors, link lecturers and lecturer-practitioners

In order to reduce the gap, the role of the link lecturer, or similar roles such as the lecturer-practitioner where there is a direct link between clinical practice and education, appear to be very well accepted and implemented. The link lecturer or lecturer-practitioner is a permanent member of the teaching staff, regularly visiting and working directly with mentees and therefore reducing any identified gaps between theory and practice. The link lecturer supports academic knowledge, is up-to-date with current, local clinical practice and maintains a permanent link between the theory providers and practice. The link lecturer model appears to work more effectively in some areas, such as the acute sector, although there is also evidence to suggest that it can potentially be a disruptive influence; a teacher doing clinicians' work can upset the daily management in the clinical area. Clearly, there will always be advantages and disadvantages to any model of mentor practice and it is often a case of achieving a balance appropriate to each clinical area.

The traditional apprenticeship approach of "see one, do one, teach one", is still in existence. Previously popular in medicine, although thankfully beginning to disappear, this is a good example of how theory–practice gaps can develop. Mentees who are taught techniques and skills poorly will repeat this performance and may go on to teach this skill again to others, so the cycle will be repeated, with potentially detrimental effects to the patient. Senior mentees may identify that the skill is incorrect and make amends; but a more junior mentee may not have the knowledge and/or expertise to be able to identify poor practice. If the mentee is then assessed on this skill by a mentor or assessor there is clearly a much higher likelihood of skill failure. Mentors themselves need to be adequately prepared for teaching, practice and assessment and this not only refers to the clinical aspect, but also to teaching and learning methods that are appropriate for the skill in question.

Therefore, effective teaching tutors/lecturer-practitioners need to be:

- Up-to-date.
- Knowledgeable.
- Proficient at the skill in question.
- Possess good teaching and assessment skills.

Similar to Benner's (2001) "know that" and "know how", Carr (2004) suggested that clinical practice is an intentional activity that has its own conceptual framework. This type of theory is not something that is applied to practice, but rather is implicit in practice. Without this theory, clinical practice becomes meaningless and random. This internal "implicit" theory demonstrates that it is possible to ride a bike without having the explicit (or external) theory of bike riding, or Benner's "know that". Similarly, paramedics will implicitly be able to cannulate a patient without thinking about the process involved – it is embedded in their subconscious.

Assessment

The word "assess" originates from the Latin "*assidere*" which means to "sit by or aside". It can also refer to deciding the worth or value of something, so the term assessment could be interpreted as meaning "staying with someone to determine the value of his or her clinical skill".

Assessment is about making a judgement about mentees, their progress and their competence, to assess their cognitive, psychomotor and affective domains of learning (Hand, 2006). There are many reasons why we assess students. The Quality Assurance Agency monitors and sets standards for UK higher education institutions and defines assessment in higher education as "any processes that appraise an individual's knowledge, understanding, abilities or skills" (Quality Assurance Agency, 2006: 4). Therefore assessment determines a mark or grade for a mentee's performance and promotes mentee learning by providing feedback to improve performance. Assessment of learning generally occurs at the conclusion of a period of learning. Genesee and Upshur (1996) suggested there were four elements to the rationale for assessments.

- Evaluation.
- Collection of information.
- Interpretation of information.
- Decision-making.

These four elements should remain the central tenets of the assessment process, regardless of the assessment method undertaken. There are a variety of assessment methods, which will be outlined below but assessments are in general either formative or summative, each serving a specific purpose.

Formative assessments

Formative assessments are usually undertaken during a programme of learning and are aimed at providing feedback to assist students in improving their clinical and professional performance. Formative assessments aim to deepen the student's understanding of the learning outcomes; any grades awarded do not contribute to the final grade or award of the programme.

Formative assessments can take a number of forms, such as a written document, for example a quiz, short answer questions or as part of a practical assessment such as an objective structured clinical examination (OSCE). Formative assessments are assessments for learning, providing feedback that aids students and their assessors/ mentors in ensuring that the programme learning outcomes are being met.

Summative assessments

Summative assessments may or may not include feedback and the key distinction between summative and formative assessments is that any grades awarded in summative assessments count towards the final overall grade for the programme. This grade will indicate performance against the standards set for the assessment and can either be part of in-course assessment or assessment at the end of a course or module. Summative assessments are therefore assessments of learning and are intended to measure learning outcomes and report those outcomes to students and their assessors/mentors.

The educational researcher, Robert Stake, explains the difference between formative and summative assessment using the following analogy:

> When the cook tastes the soup, that's formative. When the guests taste the soup, that's summative.
>
> (Stake cited in Scriven, 1991)

Informal assessments

Informal assessments are less structured and may include observation, inventories, checklists, performance and portfolio assessments, participation, peer and self-evaluation, and discussion. They are usually part of formative assessments.

Formal assessments

Formal assessments are by their nature more structured, for example written

117

exam papers, multiple choice questions (MCQs), or OSCEs and are usually, although not exclusively, an aspect of summative assessments.

Objective assessments

Objective assessments have a single correct answer, such as true/false questions, MCQs, extended matched questions (EMQs), multiple-response and matching questions. Online assessment is a popular method for conducting objective assessment since this is relatively easy to administer and grade, with immediate feedback of results.

Subjective assessments

Subjective assessments are questions that may have more than one correct answer or have more than one way of expressing the correct answer. Subjective assessments include assignments, reflective portfolios, learning journals and short answer questions.

It could be argued that there is no such thing as an objective assessment, since there is a degree of subjectivity involved in any assessment. All assessments are arguably created with inherent biases built into decisions regarding relevant subject matter and content, as well as cultural (including class, ethnic, and gender) biases. However, as discussed later, every effort is made to ensure that all assessments are as objective as possible.

Continuous assessment

Continuous assessment is a series of planned assessments of student achievement throughout the duration of the placement, usually against identified learning outcomes. Skills and competencies are monitored daily and, as previously seen in relation to clinical supervision, this can have advantages and disadvantages. Continuous assessment is advantageous in assisting in developing confidence and ensuring that mentees are aware of their development. Disadvantages include the fact that any assessment is only as good as the assessor undertaking it and the constant scrutiny may feel threatening to some mentees (Hand, 2006).

Reliability and validity

When it comes to assessing knowledge, mentors need to ensure that assessments have both high reliability and validity. The majority of higher education institution programmes from which students will require mentoring will have been validated, usually against the Health Professions Council Standards of Education and Training (Health Professions Council, 2009). Therefore the reliability and validity of the programme's assessment should, in theory at least, have already been explored and defined. In general high quality assessments are those with high levels of both reliability and validity.

Reliability

Reliability relates to the consistency of an assessment; a reliable assessment is one that consistently achieves the same results with the same (or a similar) cohort of students. Various factors affect reliability in assessments, such as ambiguous questions or standards and vague grading instructions or criteria. A good assessment is both reliable and valid, however in practice, an assessment is rarely totally valid or totally reliable. Similar to a ruler that is marked incorrectly, it will always give the same (but incorrect) measurement, so it can be said to be very reliable, but not very valid.

Validity

A valid assessment is one that measures what it is intended to measure, so for example, it would not be valid to assess infection control skills through a written assessment. A more valid method would be by demonstrating the skill of effective hand-washing and aseptic technique in wound care as well as assessing underpinning theories of microbial transfer. It can be compared with asking random individuals to tell the time without looking at a clock or watch. The answers will vary between individuals but the average answer is probably close to the actual time.

Practical examples of assessments

Practice-based assessments

Practice-based assessments are probably the core assessment type that you will be performing as a mentor. Practice-based assessments usually focus on reflective-based assessments and case studies. Although there are others available, this chapter focuses on these two types of assessment as they appear most suited to urgent care practice.

Reflective-based assessments

Reflective-based assessments can be used formatively and summatively. Formatively they can be used to assess the mentees' progress to date, providing feedback on learning and knowledge development. They can be also used summatively and are perhaps best recognised in the form of an academic assignment. Reflective-based assessments are based on recognised reflective practice frameworks.

Reflective-Based Assessment Sheet		
Gibb's Cycle	*Key facts*	*Evidence*
Description Give a brief overview of the incident		
Feelings What you were feeling and thinking at the time of the incident?		
Evaluation What was good and bad about the incident?		
Analysis What was the trigger, what knowledge were you missing, what assumptions were challenged?		
Conclusion Summarise the incident		
Action Plan How would you handle the incident if it occurred again?		

Figure 5.1. Reflective-based assessment sheet using the Gibbs Reflective Cycle.

As a formative assessment tool, reflective-based assessments are useful when the mentee is having a problem, either with a specific patient or a clinical skill. It is useful to encourage the mentee to outline a specific incident or event using a reflective-based assessment sheet (see example in *Figure 5.1*). This forms a basis for encouraging the student to talk through some of the issues and can be used for mentee discussion using the Gibbs Reflective Cycle (see *Chapter 6* for a further description of the Gibbs Cycle) (Gibbs, 1988).

The key point to reflective-based assessments is that there is evidence of further learning and analysis having taken place and any previously held beliefs and assumptions might have been challenged. The mentee will need to demonstrate evidence of supporting information, but it is a useful tool for a struggling mentee. For a summative assessment, students in higher education institutions need to complete a reflective-based assignment and any critical incident from practice can form the basis of their assignment.

Case studies

Case studies are useful learning tools, since, in addition to aiding assessment, they can be utilised as an assessment methodology. Case studies are often used as a method of focusing on a specific clinical condition and, by encouraging mentees to identify a specific patient problem, they learn through applying theory to practice, linking cognitive and psychomotor skills. For example, the mentee has been called to a Mrs Smith who has been found collapsed with a suspected stroke. Mrs Smith is subsequently diagnosed as suffering from hyperglycaemia due to undiagnosed diabetes mellitus. Researching and exploring both clinical conditions, their presenting features, aetiology and treatments assists in ensuring that learning is more realistic and related to clinical practice. This anchors mentees' experience and improves their knowledge for future cases.

Case studies differ from reflective practice in that they do not require the student to undertake any further analysis of the incident. In case studies, unlike reflective practice, there is no requirement for students to provide their own thoughts. The student may be requested to provide evidence for their discussion, such as the latest clinical guidelines, for example, but there is no remit to discuss how this has developed their learning, which is an implicit aspect of reflective practice. Case studies are useful for junior students or students new to academic study who are not familiar or comfortable with reflective practice.

The struggling student

Some students may struggle at some stage during a programme of learning. This is due to a variety of reasons but frequently involves juggling education and clinical practice with part-time programmes that never seem to feel part-time. Paramedics and nurses accessing academic programmes for the first time often lack the required study skills for adult-based and self-directed learning and will require additional support. The development of online programmes offer a solution in relation to accessing a course at a distant higher education institution, although this itself can bring challenges in terms of lack of face-to-face contact. Blended programmes offer a combination of traditional face-to-face contact with lectures and seminar groups in addition to online learning. However there is a degree of self-direction and organisation required in both approaches.

Students may also struggle with personal and home life difficulties, with some often away from home for the first time, particularly those on full-time undergraduate programmes. Lack of their usual coping framework can exacerbate any existing problems on the programme or in the learning environment. Managing students struggling in clinical placements usually falls to the mentor and ways to handle this are discussed below. A personal tutor who is able to provide pastoral support should manage students with any personal issues.

Professional guidance for mentors

It may not always be immediately obvious if a mentee is not progressing well or failing in a placement, particularly if a mentor is not working on a frequent basis with the mentee. Mentees can display a range of behaviours that are indicative of having difficulties. Maloney et al (1997) suggested that mentors should observe for the following behaviours:

- Inconsistent clinical performance.
- Not responding appropriately to constructive feedback.
- Poor preparation and organisational skills.
- Limited interactions or poor communication skills.
- Failure to adhere to local policy/protocol.
- Continual poor health; feeling depressed, angry, uncommitted, withdrawn, sad, emotionally unstable, tired or listless.

Other more specific and perhaps more explicit problematic behaviour includes attending work inappropriately dressed, e.g. wearing inappropriate jewellery, such as facial piercings; having body odour; being consistently late for shifts or not contacting the placement in event of sickness/delay; displaying insensitivity to patients and/or their relatives either in person or on the telephone; or abruptness or rudeness to other members of staff.

Whilst the Health Professions Council offers little guidance for mentors, the Royal College of Nursing has developed a Toolkit for Mentors that has useful suggestions for managing a struggling or failing student (Royal College of Nursing, 2007). Struggling students or mentees represent a real challenge for mentors; the majority of mentees perform very well, but a failing student can be stressful for mentor and mentee alike. Coping strategies for managing failing students include the following:

- Meet with the student as soon as possible to discuss the issue(s) – ensure the student is aware of the reason for the meeting.
- Discuss the situation with the student honestly and openly – students may be unaware that they are not succeeding.
- Facilitate a self-assessment to help the student identify existing knowledge and any knowledge gaps – assist in identifying sources of literature to improve knowledge/skills.
- Discuss the situation with the relevant higher education institution contact, clinical placement facilitator, practice facilitator, etc. so that you, as mentor, and the student have independent support available.

- Form a realistic action plan to address the issues and set realistic deadlines that the student understands.
- Continue to work closely with the student.
- Arrange for student to work with other mentors to ensure equity and fairness.
- Make provision for additional support or opportunities to improve within any practice areas that the student may require.
- Document weekly progress reports during this period.
- Keep contemporaneous and careful notes of all discussions and incidents and share these with the student where appropriate with joint signatures.
- Refer to and work within any other higher education institution guidelines in this area.

Failing to fail

Several research studies have highlighted the phenomenon of "failing to fail" mentees who demonstrate a lack of clinical competence in the clinical setting (Duffy and Scott, 1998; Duffy, 2003; Sharples and Kelly, 2007; Rutkowski, 2007). Several reasons were highlighted in these studies, such as allowing the personal problems of students to influence the mentor's decision.

Duffy's report (2003) for the Nursing and Midwifery Council explored this issue further by researching mentors' and lecturers' experiences regarding this issue and why some student nurses were allowed to pass clinical assessments without having demonstrated sufficient competence. Whilst this study related to nursing practice the issues are generic and therefore applicable to paramedic students. Duffy identified three key dilemmas that influenced student assessment. These were existing problems, failing theory rather than practice, and differing agendas, which are discussed below.

First, the study revealed that clinical staff were often aware that students had not been performing for some considerable time but were reluctant to put "pen to paper". This subsequently created significant frustration, even anger, in other mentors who then had to fail the student, often at an advanced stage of the programme.

Second, Duffy discovered an anomaly between the number of students failing theory and the numbers failing practice assessments. A greater number of students failed their theoretical assessment, such as an assignment, than their practice or clinical assessment. One of the possible reasons for this discrepancy was that the tool to assess the clinical skills was faulty – being too subjective and with no one validated tool used for clinical practice. A Scottish study by Norman et al (2002) on the validity and reliability of competence assessment tools concluded that there was "little or no relationship" between most of the clinical competence assessment methods that were utilised in practice (Norman et al, 2002:142). The research team recommended a multi-method approach to assessment of clinical competence.

Finally, Duffy's study also highlighted the differing agendas between the higher education institution and the clinical placement with respondents reporting that the higher education institutions did not value the practice elements of education. Some study respondents reported that students were often failing to attend theoretical sessions. This was not appropriately managed by the higher education institutions who contributed to poor professional behaviour and also failed to address high attrition rates.

Inconsistent mentorship

Although an uncomfortable topic, it is worth addressing the issue of the inconsistent mentor. While students undoubtedly fail in practice or "fail to be failed", the role of a poor mentor can compound these factors further. Mentors should be recognised professionals and experts in their field. They are often "looked up to" by students and good supportive working relationships generally develop. Dysfunction occurs when the relationship is not working for one or both parties. Scandura (1998) identified a number of potential problems that can occur, including:

- Destructive relationships – characterised by jealousy, with the mentor stifling the development of the student.
- Dependency and suffocation.
- Lack of support, or the mentor has unrealistic expectations.

As can be seen negative personal interactions can prevent students attaining their goals.

Conclusion

Mentorship has been a key element of healthcare practice for a number of years. This chapter has provided an overview of some definitions of mentorship, outlining the preparation and key skills of the mentor. The issue of competence and performance of students in practice has been addressed in relation to the theory–practice gap. Some solutions have been suggested by which to close this "gap". The issue of assessments, including different approaches to assessment, with some examples of assessment in relation to practice have been explored.

The task of mentoring is usually an additional role that practitioners adopt, sometimes with little negotiation, support or preparation in addition to an already busy clinical role. This chapter has attempted to address some of the key issues in mentoring students – whether the students are studying as part of a training course or are undergraduates from a higher education institution programme. In many respects, the professional background and the training or educational preparation of the student is irrelevant. Mentoring healthcare students requires a professional, experienced mentor who understands the key elements to developing a successful, supportive relationship with their mentee.

References

Benner P (2001) *From Novice to Expert: Excellence and power in clinical nursing practice* (Commemorative Edn). London, Sydney: Prentice Hall

Black H, Wolf A (Eds) (1990) *Knowledge and competence - Current issues in Training and Education*. Careers and Occupational Information Centre. London: HMSO

Carr SJ (2004) Assessing clinical competency in medical senior house officers: How and why should they do it? *Postgraduate Medical Journal* **80**(940): 63–6

Clements R, Mackenzie R (2005) Competence in prehospital care: Evolving concepts. *Emergency Medicine Journal* **22**(7): 516–19

Corlett J (2000) The perceptions of nurse teachers, student nurses and preceptors of the theory–practice gap in nurse education. *Nurse Education Today* **20**(6): 499–505

Darling LAW (1984) What do nurses want in a mentor? *Journal of Nursing Administration* **14**(10): 42–4

DH (2003) *AHP project: Demonstrating competence through CPD. Evaluation of the pilot exercise August 2003* (Draft document). London: HMSO

Donovan J (1990) The concept and role of mentor. *Nurse Education Today*. **10**(4): 294–8

Dreyfus H, Dreyfus S (2000) *Mind over machine. The power of human intuition and expertise in the era of the computer*. New York: Free Press

Duffy K (2003) *Failing students: A qualitative study of factors that influence the decisions regarding assessment of students' competence in practice*. Glasgow: Glasgow Caledonian University

Duffy K, Scott PA (1998) Viewing an old issue through a new lens: A critical theory insight into the education–practice gap. *Nurse Education Today* **18**(3):183–9.

Genesee F, Upshur J (1996). *Classroom-based evaluation in second language education*. Cambridge: Cambridge University Press

Gibbs G (1988) *Learning by doing: A guide to teaching and learning methods*. Further Education Unit. Oxford: Oxford Polytechnic

Girot EA (1993) Assessment of competence in clinical practice: A phenomenological approach. *Journal of Advanced Nursing* **18**(1): 114–9

Gray MA, Smith LN (2000) The qualities if an effective mentor from the student nurse's perspective: Findings from a longitudinal qualitative study. *Journal of Advanced Nursing* **32**(6): 1542–9

Hagerty B (1986) A second look at mentors. *Nursing Outlook* **34**(1): 1624

Hand H (2006) Assessment of learning in clinical practice. *Nursing Standard* **21**(4): 48–56

Health Professions Council (2009). *Standards of education and training*. London: HPC

Lakasing E, Francis H (2005) The crisis in student mentorship. *Primary Health Care* **15**(4): 40–1

Lankshear A (1990) Failure to fail: The teacher's dilemma. *Nursing Standard* **4**(20): 35–7

Loads D, Brown M, McKenzie K, Powell H (2006) Developing mentorship through collaboration. *Learning Disability Practice* **9**(3): 16–8

Maloney D, Carmody D, Nemeth E (1997) Students experiencing problems learning in the clinical setting. In McAllister L, Lincoln M, McLeod S, Maloney D (Eds) *Facilitating learning in clinical settings* (pp 185–213). Cheltenham: Stanley Thornes

Norman IJ, Watson R, Murrells T, Calman L, Redfern S (2002) The validity and reliability of methods to assess the competence to practise of pre-registration nursing and midwifery students. *International Journal of Nursing Studies* **39**(2): 133–45

Nursing & Midwifery Council (2008) *Standards to Support Learning and Assessment in Practice*. London. NMC

Price B (2006) Addressing problematic behaviour in learners. *Nursing Standard* **20**(40): 47–8

Quality Assurance Agency for Higher Education (2006) *Code of practice for the assurance of academic quality and standards in higher education. Section 6: Assessment of students*. Gloucester: QAA

Quality Assurance Agency (2010) *Evaluation of the academic infrastructure: A QAA discussion paper*. Gloucester: QAA

Royal College of Nursing (2007) *Guidance for mentors of nursing students and midwives* An RCN toolkit. London: RCN

Rutkowski K (2007) Failure to fail: Assessing nursing students' competence during practice. *Nursing Standard* **22**(13): 35–40

Scandura TA (1998) Dysfunctional mentoring relationships and outcomes. *Journal of Management* **24**(3): 449–67

Scriven M (1991). *Evaluation thesaurus*. (4th Edn.) Newbury Park, CA: Sage Publications

Sharples K, Kelly D (2007) Supporting mentors in practice. *Nursing Standard*

21(39): 44–7

While AE (1994) Competence versus performance: Which is more important? *Journal of Advanced Nursing* **20**(3): 525–31

CHAPTER 6

Reflective practice

This chapter presents an overview of reflective practice. The rationale for presenting a brief synopsis is largely for paramedic readers; nurses have a much longer history in relation to using and adopting reflective practice for their learning and development.

Definitions of reflective practice

Reflective practice can be defined as:

> ... the complex and deliberate process of thinking about and interpreting experience in order to learn from it ...
>
> (Getliffe, 1996: 362)

There are various definitions and readers should select a definition that suits their needs and context. Reflective practice is essentially in two parts – reflection and practice. Reflection involves taking a mirror and looking, usually retrospectively, at clinical practice. Practice involves the clinical activity of the healthcare professional, whether in a clinical, educational or managerial role.

Example of reflective practice

Mezirow (1990) stated that reflection allows a practitioner to challenge any previously held beliefs, values or ideals and apply these in a problem-solving approach to a "critical" incident. A critical incident is one that stands out to the practitioner for a specific reason and does not necessarily relate to a critically ill or injured patient. In fact, some of the best reflective practice assignments relate to apparently trivial events.

One example is a paramedic emergency care practitioner student who reflected on a patient consultation in "Minors" in an emergency department. A single mother of three young children presented with a painful wrist following a fall, and was subsequently diagnosed with a scaphoid fracture. When informed of the diagnosis and the plaster cast treatment, she promptly burst into tears, questioning the student on how she was supposed to cope with three young children with her dominant arm immobilised in plaster for several weeks. The student's assignment focused on the issue of how such a seemingly minor injury, from the practitioner's perspective, was actually a major injury in terms of the patient and her ability to manage at home with a young family.

Reflective practitioners

Reflective practitioners need to be intent on entering into a learning cycle. By drawing on past experiences they can gain insight to generate new knowledge. Within the nursing profession, the work of Schön (1983) has been influential on reflective practice. Action that is based on the reflection of past experience, values and beliefs form the basis of Schön's theory of reflection-*in*-action, where the practitioner recognises a problem and uses his or her previous experience to act on it. By contrast reflection-*on*-action is aimed at retrospectively analysing and interpreting an event and applying new knowledge gained to any similar future situations.

Reflective learning

Reflective learning is a process where the examination and exploration of an issue of concern, triggered by a specific experience, is clarified into some form of meaning, thereby changing the individual's perspective (Boyd and Fales, 1983). Reflective learning has been used in the nursing, midwifery and health visiting professions to provide a framework for reviewing and analysing clinical incidents. It is important to have a good understanding and working knowledge of reflective practice before facilitating the learning of students. There are a number of reflective practice models, which are useful in assisting both practitioners and students in clinical placements and which are also useful for theoretical summative assessment, such as reflective practice assignments.

Reflective practice assignments

All the reflective practice models have some common key elements, and choice is largely a case of personal preference. When using reflective practice models for assignments and for reflective-based assessments it is important to anonymise all patient identifiable information and make a reference regarding confidentiality. It is also good practice to ensure that reference is made to the patient's consent for the practitioner's examination or assessment. Although similar to case studies, in that reflective practice focuses on specific patients, it may not necessarily focus on the clinical aspect of a scenario but rather on the specific rationale for why the student/practitioner selected that particular patient or critical incident.

The rationale for selecting a specific incident is usually because the patient challenged a previously held belief, or perhaps the patient's own understanding or knowledge of a specific aspect of his or her condition, presentation or response to treatment, such as the example referred to earlier, challenges the practitioner. As such, reflective practice is often written up in the first person as opposed to the third person, the latter being common in most academic assignments.

Some assignments are worthy of publication and are welcomed as there is a limited base of paramedic reflective practice assignments, and students find these really useful. However there are distinct differences between writing up assignments and writing academic articles for publication and it is always worth consulting the intended journal for supporting advice and guidance.

Reflective practice models

There are a number of reflective practice models and any one of these models can be utilised as a framework for practice or an assignment; it is a case of selecting the model that is most appropriate. Four commonly used reflective practice models are:

- The Gibbs Reflective Cycle.
- The Atkins and Murphy Model.
- The Johns Model of Structured Reflection.
- Boud et al's What, Now What, So What Model.

Gibbs (1988) Reflective Cycle

The Gibbs Reflective Cycle is probably the most well-known reflective practice model. This is largely because it is a relatively easy model to understand and apply making it popular with students new to reflective practice or academic study. There are six elements to the Gibbs Cycle: description, feelings, evaluation, analysis, conclusion and action plan, as seen in *Figure 6.1*.

Description
As in any assignment, a description of the incident as a form of introduction to the "story" is required. The description should act as a "verbal snapshot" or a précis of the incident and is usually two to three paragraphs in length. It provides an overview of the events leading up to the incident, the incident itself and any outcomes. Perhaps the best way of approaching this section is to imagine writing a short confidential report to your line manager outlining an untoward event.

Feelings
This section frequently generates the most derision – paramedics claim not to "do" feelings. However it does not require a deep analytical thesis on your

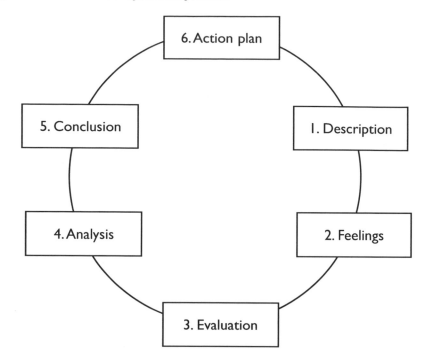

Figure 5.2. The Gibbs Reflective Cycle.

choice of incident, it simply requires the inclusion of any thoughts and feelings at the time of the incident. For example, this could be a feeling of isolation when you are presented with an unconscious motorcyclist in the middle of country lane on a dark, wet night with no available medical help for 15 minutes; or a feeling of helplessness or frustration when a patient with end-of-life care is in intractable pain, which you are unable to alleviate despite your best efforts, and there is no available GP with whom to discuss the case.

Feelings are generally "one-worders" – i.e. panic, fright, isolation, fear, happy, etc. They are usually easy to recall and they assist the practitioner in identifying why this incident was important, offering an opportunity for further explanation. The feelings section should be fairly short; sometimes students assume that they are required to write an in-depth account of their innermost thoughts – this in not the case.

Evaluation

The key feature of this section is to outline what was good and bad about the incident. For example, this might be whether the room/area was very noisy making it difficult to hear or talk to the patient. Did you feel rushed to complete your assessment or examination of the patient? Was there a talkative relative who kept answering the questions you were asking the patient? Did the examination/ consultation go well? Did you feel that there was something the patient/relative was not telling you? Again this is a relatively short section and assists in the understanding of why the incident was pertinent to the practitioner.

Analysis

This is the real nitty-gritty of reflection and should be the longest section of the assignment. It is also the most challenging since it involves reviewing your actions or the actions of others "under a microscope". Analysis allows exploration of the individual components of an incident, identifying any existing knowledge, challenging assumptions or beliefs and exploring any alternatives.

In reflective practice, practitioners may well be critical of themselves or others. However this should be constructive criticism and in line with the objective approach taken throughout the assignment. The practitioner is required to reference appropriate literature, so if, for example, the incident raised an issue of communication, then literature referring to communication theories need to be included. This is essential in reflective practice, since practitioners are required to support their learning and challenge values and beliefs with evidence.

Conclusion

The conclusion provides a short summary of the incident, summarising the key points in the text, similar to a conclusion in an assignment or the end of a story.

Action plan

The action plan focuses on presenting any new knowledge gained from this particular incident, in the light of how the practitioner would manage a similar incident in the future. It may be difficult to state definitively how you might address an identical situation, since it could be argued that all situations vary slightly. However the main aim of this section is to highlight specific areas or points that have changed as a result of the reflective practice exercise and include any new knowledge or learning.

Atkins and Murphy (1993)

The Atkins and Murphy "model" is not actually a model. The authors undertook a literature review of the various skills that were required for reflective practice and identified some key stages in reflection. However it has subsequently been adopted as a model for reflective practice and is a useful framework. The four identified elements are description, critical analysis, synthesis and evaluation.

Description

The description section relates to the ability to recognise and recollect accurately salient events and key features of an incident, providing a comprehensive account of the situation. The practitioner should also note the awareness of any uncomfortable feelings and thoughts, as in the Gibbs Cycle. The ability to describe and write about feelings enables learning through reflection.

Critical analysis

Critical analysis involves examining the components of the incident, identifying any existing or current knowledge, challenging previously held assumptions and exploring alternatives. A critical analysis of knowledge also involves examining how relevant knowledge is to an individual incident. Similar to the analysis section of the Gibbs Cycle, reference to the appropriate literature or evidence base is required at this point to support new knowledge, challenge existing information, and perhaps begin to support an argument for a change in practice.

Synthesis

Synthesis is the integration of new and prior knowledge and its use in a creative way to problem-solve and predict likely consequences of action. This has similarities with the action plan section in the Gibbs Cycle. Synthesis represents the merging of evidence to allow new practice to either take place or be recommended.

Evaluation

Evaluation involves making a judgement about the value of something and entails the use of criteria and standards. In addition to synthesis, evaluation is invaluable in developing new perspectives in relation to the incident, although it should be noted that this differs slightly from the evaluation stage in the Gibbs Cycle. Evaluation in this model, in addition to synthesis, is invaluable in assisting the practitioner to develop new perspectives.

Johns (1991, 1994) Model of Structured Reflection

The Johns Model consists of a series of questions that aim to assist practitioners in structuring their reflective thinking in a meaningful way. The Johns Model focuses on a core question: "What information do I need access to in order to learn from this experience?" To answer this, Johns suggested that there are the following five "cue questions". (An incident is referred to as an "experience" in this model.)

Description of experience
- Phenomenon: Description of the "here and now" experience.
- Causal: What essential factors contributed to this experience?
- Context: What are the significant background factors to this experience?
- Clarifying: What are the key processes (for reflection) in the experience?

Reflection

- What was I attempting to achieve?
- Why did I intervene as I did?
- What were the consequences of my actions for:
  - Myself?
  - The patient/family?
  - For the people I work with?
- How did I feel about this experience when it was happening?
- How did the patient feel about it?
- How do I know how the patient felt about it?

Influencing factors

- What internal factors influenced my decision-making?
- What external factors influenced my decision-making?
- What sources of knowledge did/should have influenced my decision-making?

Could I have dealt better with the situation?

- What other choices did I have?
- What would be the consequences of these choices?

Learning

- How do I now feel about this experience?
- How have I made sense of the experience in light of past experiences and future practice?
- How has this experience changed my ways of knowing?

Boud, Keogh and Walker (1985) What? So What? and Now What? approach

The Boud, Keogh and Walker model focuses on three key elements that encompass the process of reflection (an incident is referred to as a situation in this model). These included:

- Returning to the situation: Recalling the salient or key events.
- Attending to feelings: Using helpful and removing unhelpful feelings.
- Evaluating experience: Re-examining the incident in the light of new knowledge.

This model is perhaps better known as the What?, So What? and Now What? approach.

What (or returning to the situation)
- is the purpose of returning to the situation?
- exactly occurred in your own words? (describe)
- did you see or do?
- was your reaction?
- did other people do, e.g. colleague, patient, relative?

So what (attending to feelings)
- were your feelings at the time?
- are your feeling now and are there differences and, if so, why?
- were the effects of what you did (or did not do)?
- "good" emerged from the incident, e.g. for yourself and others?
- troubles you about the situation (if anything)?
- were your experiences in comparison with your colleagues, etc?
- are the main reasons for feeling different from your colleagues, etc?

Now what (evaluating experience)
- are the implications for you, your colleagues, the patient, etc?
- needs to happen to alter the situation?
- are you going to do about the situation?
- happens if you decide not to alter anything?
- might you do differently if faced with a similar situation again?
- information do you need to face a similar situation again?
- are the best ways of getting further information about the situation should it arise again?

Not all of the questions need to be asked; they are there to act as a guide for the practitioner. The Boud, Keogh and Walker model is popular with junior students and students new to reflective practice as it offers a a logical, step-wise, easy-to-follow approach.

Summary

There are a number of reflective practice models that can be applied to clinical practice or assignments. Like any skill, reflective practice takes time to learn and understand and the best way of improving is simply to practise. Learning through reflection is known as reflexivity and refers to practitioners understanding and comprehending how they learn using reflective practice. In other words, by practitioners asking themselves, "What have I learnt from this incident that I could use again?"

All reflective practice models provide a framework by which to achieve this learning. They are best thought of as a coat hanger on which to hang and frame your knowledge. If knowledge, like clothes, were in a jumbled heap on the floor it does not make much sense. By hanging clothes on a hanger, or by "hanging" knowledge and experience on a framework then that knowledge will make sense and can be applied to future practice,

References

Atkins S, Murphy K (1993) Reflection: A review of the literature. *Journal of Advanced Nursing* **18**(8): 1188–92

Boud D, Keogh R, Walker D (1985) (Eds) *Reflection: Turning experience into learning*. London: Kogan Page

Boyd EM, Fales AW (1983) Reflective learning: Key to learning from experience. *Journal of Humanistic Psychology* **23**(2): 99–117

Getliffe KA (1996) An examination of the use of reflection in the assessment of practice for undergraduate nursing students. *International Journal of Nursing Studies* **33**(4): 361–74

Gibbs G (1988) *Learning by doing: A guide to teaching and learning methods*. Further Education Unit. Oxford: Oxford Polytechnic

Johns C (1991) The Burford Nursing Development Unit holistic model of nursing practice. *Journal of Advanced Nursing* **16**(9): 1090–8.

Johns C (1994) Guided reflection. In Palmer A, Burns S, Bulman C (Eds) *Reflective practice in nursing: The growth of the professional practitioner*. Oxford: Blackwell Science

Mezirow J (1990) *Fostering critical reflection in adulthood: A guide to emancipatory learning*. San Francisco: Jossey-Bass

Schön DA (1983) *The reflective practitioner*. New York: Basic Books

Section Three

Legal and ethical issues

This section provides an account of the legal issues and ethical principles in healthcare. Some key legal cases are identified in an endeavour to further highlight the most important principles in some detail and explore their application to urgent care practice. There are a number of other legal cases that are relevant to urgent clinical care, but these largely fall outside the remit of this book. Details of some are given so that readers can access them should they wish to do so.

Both chapters in this section aim to stimulate debate, encourage further reading and hopefully inspire readers to consider some of the important aspects of legal and ethical issues in relation to their specific practice within urgent care.

This Section is therefore not intended to be a definitive text on the legal and ethical issues in urgent care, but rather an overview of the core principles, with application to some of the common themes that are presented in the unique and emerging field of paramedic practice.

Chapter 7 focuses on some fundamental legal issues. Any text relating to medicolegal issues would of course not be complete without directing readers to the large numbers of excellent texts relating to the subject in medicine and nursing. However, there is a developing literature base in paramedic practice. The principles addressed here are generic and therefore applicable to both paramedic and nursing practice.

Chapter 8 is on ethical principles, with specific application to urgent care practice. It addresses the four ethical principles of autonomy, nonmaleficence, beneficence and justice. Autonomy is developed in relation to informed consent and data protection. Nonmaleficence is explored in relation to the controversy surrounding the measles, mumps and rubella vaccine, aspects of negligence, and practice guidelines. Beneficence is considered in relation to the management of pain and dignity. Finally the issue of justice is presented with further discussion of clinical guidelines in practice and the distribution of care.

CHAPTER 7

Legal issues

Setting the scene

This chapter focuses on legal issues, specifically those that relate to accountability, obligation and duty. The issue of accountability is considered in relation to the development of the paramedic practitioner role. Obligation is discussed in relation to the issue of vulnerable individuals and with particular reference to the identification and management of child maltreatment. Duty is discussed with regard to negligence in clinical care, competency and the role of the National Health Service Litigation Authority. There are of course a number of other relevant elements related to legal issues, but these three areas appear to be most relevant to urgent care.

Some key legal cases are presented in order to highlight some of the fundamental principles of these legal issues. There are numerous legal examples of cases that are relevant to this field of clinical care, and where possible, these are identified. Interested readers can access further case details via the Internet.

Accountability

The political background to the emerging field of urgent care has impacted on how the various roles have evolved, as seen with the development of the emergency care practitioner (ECP) and paramedic practitioner as discussed earlier. The subsequent shaping of clinical practice, combined with the rapid changes in the role of the practitioner in urgent care, has been as a direct result of some of the political changes both from national and wider influences. With an increasing proportion of urgent care being delivered by non-medical personnel, such as paramedics and nurses, some of the accountability issues have also changed. With increased clinical responsibility comes increased answerability. One consideration is that if the paramedic or nurse practitioner is delivering care usually provided by, or on behalf of, a doctor, then where does accountability lie?

The advancement of the role of the paramedic and nurse in urgent care, which includes the ability to undertake examination and assessment of patients, document their history, recommend and refer for ongoing treatment and prescribe a range of medications, has medico-legal implications. In some aspects of such care, the law and relevant policy has yet to catch up with practice. However, certain issues, such as paramedic prescribing, will inevitably become common practice over the next few years.

Accountability is a concept based in ethics and governance and will be considered with the two associated concepts of responsibility and liability.

Responsibility

One of the key drivers for change, specifically from the perspective of the emergency nurse practitioner or paramedic practitioner working within the emergency department, minor injuries unit or walk-in clinic is the change in junior doctor hours. The European Working Time Directive has had a significant impact, particularly in the acute sector. The Directive was derived from the Council of Europe (Department of Health, 2009) and was intended to protect the health and safety of workers in the European Union. It sets out minimum requirements of working hours, annual leave and rest breaks. The law was enacted in the UK in 1998 and since 2003, the working hours of junior doctors is limited to 56 hours per week, considerably less than they previously worked.

Whilst the Directive has no doubt improved the well-being of doctors, reducing tiredness and stress, it has not of course eliminated the need for continuous care. Many trusts responded by developing innovative models of care delivery. These have included changes to the emergency department, where the flow of patients is largely unpredictable since there is no "gate-keeping" capability, as in other sectors of healthcare. Many emergency departments adopted alternative care pathways to manage patients. Studies suggest that emergency nurse practitioners could not only undertake the clinical role of senior house officers but often out-performed them across a range of specialties. They also reduced the out of hours workload, including in specialist areas such as ophthalmology (Ezra et al, 2005).

Studies of the cost implications of the development of the nurse practitioner role revealed similar findings (Department of Health, 2006). More challenging to measure is, of course, the quality of the care provided and the patient response to the care. Some studies suggested that the ECP role was not just a cheaper alternative to traditional models of care (Skills for Health, 2007); these practitioners appeared to provide was a more holistic package of patient-centred care that was preferred by the patients (Cooper et al, 2002). Utilising ECPs to manage patients with "minor" injuries was effective and cost efficient (Cooke et al, 2002). However Richards et al (2004) concluded that delegating the management of patients with minor illness to nurses in a telephone triage system may result in an overall increase in the number of presenting problems per patient as the GPs tended to act as if the patient caseload was more challenging, due to increased prescriptions and consultations, which may then subsequently impact in changing GP's consulting behaviours.

The various role titles can lead to confusion, not least to their contributing professions, and the lack of standardisation in these roles needs addressing. The nurse practitioner role has been evident in the UK for almost two decades but there is still some degree of variation in the preparatory academic programmes. A review of the professionals themselves by Currie and Couch (2007) highlighted this further. One key issue was that of management and supervision. The seniority of these professionals often resulted in them supervising junior medical staff, which in itself created a dilemma. The boundary between medical and nursing practice has been blurring over the years, with the "ceiling" no longer being present as to the limit of nurse practitioners' practice. One respondent in the study suggested that a "homogenous core of emergency care clinicians" may evolve and that the traditional title of doctor and nurse would become obsolete (Currie and Crouch, 2007: 337).

In some urgent care settings this "homogenous urgent care practitioner" has already evolved; critical care practitioners in air ambulance and helicopter emergency medical services work very closely with their medical colleagues, forming a tight knit team, each with a range of complementary skills and competencies.

How does this additional role change affect the accountability of such practitioners? With increased responsibility comes increased accountability and the legal framework by which this is measured is not clear. During the course of this chapter, this specific issue will be addressed further since it appears fundamental to the urgent care practitioner.

Liability

In relation to liability, it is worth considering the role of the National Health Service Litigation Authority (NHSLA) in the legal functioning of the NHS. The NHSLA is a special health authority that came into existence in November 1995 in order to deal with negligence claims and to work to improve the practice and management of NHS risk. NHSLA risk management standards are available for all NHS healthcare organisations, including the acute and ambulance trusts. The standards are designed to address the organisational, clinical, and non-clinical health and safety risks associated with trusts. The NHSLA and clinical negligence will be discussed later.

From a patient or service user perspective, there are essentially two schemes under which claimants can make clinical negligence claims. These are the Clinical Negligence Scheme for Trusts handling any claims that took place on or after 1st April 1995. Membership to this scheme is voluntary, although currently all NHS trusts belong. The Existing Liabilities Scheme refers to clinical negligence claims against the NHS in England before April 1995. Initially handling lower value claims, since April 2000 all Existing Liabilities Scheme claims are handled through the NHSLA.

In relation to urgent care, one of the identified clinical risk areas for ambulance trusts, under the clinical care standard, is that of extended care practitioners. These individuals are termed "advanced practitioners" and they are capable of assessing, treating, discharging or referring patients at the scene of contact, such as in the home or workplace. They have undertaken specific training and education to enable them to respond to the first contact needs of patients accessing urgent care. The key areas for assessment were the monitoring of these practitioners in terms of their use of approved documentation and their care of patients in relation to treatments, including prescribing. Similar documentation is published for acute trusts (NHSLA, 2009/10) and their identified risk areas include clinical record keeping, consent, and medicines management amongst others, with application to the walk-in centre and minor injuries unit type settings.

Litigation and the ambulance service

Some research has been undertaken to assess claims related to urgent care, including that by Williams (2007) who undertook a review of all claims bought against ambulance services submitted to the NHSLA between 1995 and 2004. The reliability of the data is questionable since the NHSLA has only handled such claims, regardless of value, since 2002. Prior to this, claims of lower value were dealt with in-house by the appropriate trust and reporting to the NHSLA was optional between 1995 and 2002. Despite these constraints, it was estimated that 263 reported claims were brought, which included either the delayed arrival of ambulance on scene or some other form of delay. The most frequent complaint (76%) included faulty diagnosis or a medication/equipment failure; delays in response accounted for fewer than 20% of all claims.

A similar review conducted by Dobbie and Cooke (2008) identified 272 cases of litigation against ambulance trusts in the UK highlighting a 900% rise in claims between 1995 and 2004; (27%) were for lack of assistance or care. The failure or delay in admission to hospital, treatment, diagnosis or referral to hospital accounted for a combined total of 43.7% of all claims. Other claims related to incidents involving poor pain management (20.6%), fracture (9.7%), brain damage (7.7%), cardiac arrest (1.1%), and stroke (0.4%).

Potential reasons for the rise in claims is the apparent increasingly litigious nature of our society in general, with the general public having a lower tolerance level for errors and a higher expectation for standards of care. The introduction of "no win no fee" legal arrangements has increased access to legal advice, perhaps also explaining this exponential rise in the number of claimants. In the US there is tendency to practise defensive medicine or care that is the most safe but not necessarily the most efficacious. In the UK there are three identified features that impact on medical negligence claims, which include the following:

- Time taken to bring action to a conclusion.
- The cost of awards of damages (in 2008/09 there were 6080 claims of clinical negligence received by the NHSLA costing £769 million, NHSLA, 2010/11).
- Care taken by courts to operate in light of medical reality of practice and the impact on respect for the profession.

For a legal case example, see *Roe v Minister of Health* (1954).

In 1996 the Department for Constitutional Affairs published the Woolf Report which outlined reforms for the role of courts and judges in hearing medical negligence cases (medical in this context referring to any healthcare professional). Lord Woolf clearly stated that the cost of medical litigation was too high, only being accessible to patients with the support of legal aid. The costs were due to the complexity of the law and the unrealistic expectations, in some cases, of the patients in relation to their treatment. Some doctors react defensively with aggrieved patients, heightening their disappointment in what they perceive as a refused acknowledgement of their complaint and subsequent "cover up". Lord Woolf outlined a number of recommendations including the need for the education of health professionals in the legal context of health care and for the various professional bodies to clarify the responsibility of HCPs to their patients when an act of omission occurs, and in which they may have been negligent. One important recommendation was that the legal route was not always required. Many patients simply wanted the relevant person and/or organisation to apologise for their error – monetary compensation was often not their aim. At the time of the report, there was often little choice but to advise litigation, although other options were available, such as financial recourse or impartial information and advice.

The blurring of professional boundaries between the traditional nurse, paramedic and doctor role have further complicated issues. Dowling et al (1996) and latterly Buttress and Marangon (2008) explored this issue in relation to accountability. Dowling et al identified, in the early stages of nurses extending their roles, that the regulations arising between the two professional bodies of nursing and medicine raised uncertainties about the appropriate management for the clinical roles between the professions. In the late 1990s the UKCC (now the Nursing and Midwifery Council), nursing's professional body, stated that whatever role, or title, the nurse undertook, s/he was still accountable to the UKCC. The challenge arose when, if a nurse were deemed to be negligent due to some error, then to which standard would s/he be held accountable? These practitioners needed to work within their competency – a view that still held firm in the Buttress and Marangon paper. The NHS Plan (Department of Health, 2000c) acknowledged the rapid rise in the number of nurse consultants and nurse specialists who undertake roles that were previously traditionally considered to be those of the doctor. The role of the paramedic appears to be following a similar course.

Medical negligence law

In relation to the concept of accountability, the law on medical negligence has played a significant role in determining the standard of care expected. Negligence is perhaps best simply defined as the omission to do something that a reasonable person would do. However, this definition is only suitable for those activities that are open to all practitioners and there are different definitions in relation to activities that can only properly be undertaken by expert practitioners. The accepted version of this definition stems from the case highlighted below.

Bolam v Friern Hospital Management Committee

Perhaps the most frequently quoted and well-known case in relation to medical negligence is that of *Bolam v Friern Hospital Management Committee* (1957). In this case, Mr Bolam was a voluntary patient at a mental health institution, run by the Friern Hospital Management Committee. Mr Bolam agreed to undergo electro-convulsive therapy (ECT) as a treatment for mental health issues, but was not administered any relaxant drugs nor restrained during the procedure. He subsequently suffered a number of serious injuries, including a fractured acetabulum and pelvis. He subsequently sued Friern Hospital Management Committee for compensation, claiming that they were negligent for not issuing relaxants, for not restraining him and for not warning him regarding the risks involved. The risk of a fractured acetabulum was accepted as a 1:10000 and, at this time, medical opinion was divided, with some doctors warning of fracture risk whilst others not, in the belief that this would confuse the patient who was, by definition, already suffering from mental health problems.

At the time, the management and use of ECT was varied. It had been developed in several centres and there were varying views on its management with some doctors favouring the use of therapeutic relaxants, some using restraint, whilst others thought that neither was helpful. The judge in this case took the view that it was "inappropriate" to choose between these differing bodies of opinion and directed the jury that "a doctor is not guilty of negligence if he has acted in accordance with a practice accepted as proper by a responsible body of medical men skilled in that particular art". In the Bolam case, this raised two questions; first, was the information provided accurate and appropriate, and second, was the treatment properly managed? The jury in this case decided that there had been no negligence.

The Bolam Test is the English tort law case (a tort law is a body of law that addresses and remedies civil wrongs) that outlines the rules for assessing the appropriate standards of reasonable care in negligence cases involving skilled professionals, such as doctors. In other words, the Bolam Test states:

If a doctor reaches the standard of a responsible body of medical opinion, he is not negligent.

Where defendants (practitioners) represent themselves as having more than average skills and abilities, this test expects standards that must be in accordance with a responsible body of opinion, even if others differ in opinion. The Bolam Test followed the rather oddly titled Clapham Omnibus Test that states:

Where you get a situation which involves the use of some special skill or competence, then the test as to whether there has been negligence is not the test of the man on the top of a Clapham omnibus, because he has not got this special skill.

The key aspect of the Clapham Omnibus Test is that the defendant does not have a special or particular skill – it is the skill expected of the average practitioner in that particular clinical field.

The rules for assessing the appropriate standards of reasonable care in negligence cases are that where the skilled professional has represented him or herself as having more than average skills these are in accordance with a responsible body of opinion, even if others differ in their opinion. As such, if a doctor reaches the standard of a responsible body of medical opinion, s/he is not negligent.

The question is raised as to whether these "tests" could be applied to allied healthcare professionals, specifically those with additional skills and expertise, who could potentially be sued for negligence – will the Bolam and Clapham Omnibus Tests apply to them?

Obligation

The concept of obligation is presented here in relation to the management of vulnerable patients. An obligation is defined as a requirement to take some course of action and whether this action is legal or moral and in relation to clinical practice. The focus in this chapter is on the legal and moral obligations of the urgent care practitioner managing patients from vulnerable groups. Vulnerable groups, including adults and children, frequently present in the urgent and pre-hospital care setting and the importance of whose needs can be sometimes be overlooked.

Vulnerable adults

A vulnerable adult is defined as "a person aged 18 years or over, who is in receipt of, or may be in need of, community care services by reason of mental or other disability, age or illness and who is or may be unable to take care of him/herself or unable to protect him/herself against significant harm or exploitation" (Department of Health, 2000a: 8–9).

The Protection of Vulnerable Adults scheme was initially implemented to safeguard those at risk from maltreatment from care staff. The Bichard Inquiry Report (2004) was published following the murder of Holly Wells and Jessica Chapman in Soham, Cambridgeshire in 2002, by Ian Huntley. Whilst Huntley had come to the attention of Humberside Police in relation to a number of alleged sexual offences, this information was not revealed during a vetting check for the school in which he worked and where Holly and Jessica were pupils. The Bichard Inquiry Report (2004) reviewed the child protection procedures in Humberside Police and Cambridgeshire Constabulary and it particularly focused on the effectiveness of relevant intelligence-based record keeping and the vetting practices and also the information sharing, or lack of it, between agencies. The Report made a number of recommendations on matters of local and national relevance, particularly in relation to record keeping and vetting practices.

The Government adopted many of the recommendations from the Bichard Inquiry Report and subsequently published the Safeguarding Vulnerable Groups Act (OPSI, 2006), which came into force in 2009. The purpose of the Act was to minimise harm to children and vulnerable adults and to strengthen the existing arrangements under the Protection of Children Act (OPSI, 1999). One of the fundamental issues highlighted in the Bichard Inquiry was the lack of a single agency to assess the suitability of individuals, and the Independent Safeguarding Authority was formed to fulfil this role. This Act also addressed a range of activities, relevant to urgent care, that provided the opportunity for close contact with children, such as the "frequent and intensive contact with children or vulnerable adults in a place such as a hospital, clinic or school" (Griffith and Tengnah, 2009: 310).

From October 2009, employers and managers of organisations working with vulnerable groups, such as ambulance and acute trust staff, now have a duty to comply with the new law. Part of this duty includes referral to the Independent Safeguarding Authority of dismissals for conduct that harms, or poses a risk of harm to children or vulnerable adults, with penalties for non-compliance, in addition to their existing reporting procedures in such circumstances.

Vulnerable children

Every week, in the UK, approximately four children are killed at the hands of another person, often known to the child (Ofsted, 2008). Reference to child maltreatment will undoubtedly bring to mind the cases of Victoria Climbié and, more recently, Peter Connelly. The Victoria Climbié Inquiry (Laming, 2003) runs to over 400 pages and makes a total of 108 recommendations for the health, emergency and social services. For healthcare, the Inquiry suggested that for any child admitted to hospital with suspected deliberate harm, the nursing care plan must take full account of this diagnosis (Recommendation 64) and the doctor or nurse admitting the child must inquire about previous admissions (Recommendation 73). Other recommendations are that any child admitted to hospital about whom there are concerns about deliberate harm must receive a comprehensive and fully documented physical examination within 24 hours of admission, except when doing so would, in the opinion of the examining doctor, compromise the child's care or the child's physical and emotional well-being (Recommendation 74).

Maltreatment

Of the approximately 9.6 million children and young people aged 16 years and under in England, Cawson (2002) reported that 7% would experience serious physical maltreatment at the hands of their parents or carers during childhood and 4% would experience sexual maltreatment.

Other countries in the UK report similar findings; in Scotland there were 6600 children referred for child protection issues during 2000–2001 and there were 4330 calls to Childline Scotland (Scottish Executive, 1999). In Northern Ireland, under 16-year-olds account for 22% of the population, with almost 2000 being on the Child Protection Register and this number is steadily increasing (NSPCC, 2008). In Wales 2500 children were on the Child Protection Register as of 2009 (NSPCC, 2009). In addition there are probably many more unreported and unrecognised cases of child maltreatment in the community.

The National Society for the Prevention of Cruelty to Children (NSPCC) claims that child maltreatment is inherently difficult to define because children can be harmed in many different ways other than physically, sexually or emotionally. Maltreatment can often be interlinked and overlapping, making it difficult to estimate the total number of maltreated children (NSPCC, 2009). The NSPCC is the only UK charity to be granted statutory powers under the 1989 Children Act permitting it to apply for care and supervision orders for children deemed at risk. Although there are limited data available on the financial implications of maltreatment either in the short or long term, in 1996 the annual cost in the UK was estimated to be £735 million (Department of Health, 1996).

By spring of 2008, almost 36000 children and young people were on child protection registers in Wales, Northern Ireland and Scotland, or the subject of a child protection plan in England, because of suffering maltreatment or being at risk of maltreatment. For the 12 months to March 2009, over 500000 referrals were made to all social services for children deemed "at risk", reported by healthcare professionals, teachers, voluntary workers, friends, family or neighbours. Many more children in similar situations probably go unnoticed or unreported and practitioners in urgent care, who are often in frequent contact with children, are in a position to make a real difference by bringing a child that is suffering to the notice of those who can help.

In a literature review of studies using screening tests to detect physical abuse in children attending UK emergency departments from 1974 to 2004, Woodman et al (2008) revealed that 66 of the studies were of poor quality. Their review suggested that child maltreatment affects 1 in 11 children in the UK annually, accounting for approximately 1% of all emergency department attendances. This suggested that physical abuse was frequently overlooked in children attending emergency departments, as the clinical screening tests were poorly quantified. The paper concluded that there was "no evidence to suggest that any test was highly predictive of physical abuse" (Woodman et al, 2008: 3).

A further study (Sidebotham et al, 2007) of the protocols adopted by emergency departments to identify and manage child maltreatment demonstrated a lack of consistency in approach. The authors recommended that a good standard of guidelines should be made available for emergency departments. Children aged one year and under were more likely to be severely injured than older children and even the presence of an emergency department community liaison nurse did not appear to improve the performance of the screening test, resulting in only approximately 50% of abused children being referred to social services. The authors also noted that the poor quality of the data played a role in their findings, recommending that improved clinical screening was probably more useful than protocols aimed at improving the detection of child maltreatment.

Kaye et al (2009) identified similar results in their study, prompted by the discrepancy in the actual and expected number of child protection referrals from the emergency department based on local demographics. Their study also highlighted that children with parents suffering from mental illness were considered specifically at risk of maltreatment.

Maltreatment, whether in children or adults, is one of the most common reasons for vulnerable individuals to access urgent care. Maltreatment often occurs in people's own homes so paramedics are ideally placed to identify it since they are in the unique position of consulting with patients in their homes or places of residence and can witness at first hand what may be missed by another professional in a hospital setting.

Maltreatment is defined as

> *... a single act or repeated acts ... it may be physical, verbal or psychological. It may be an act of neglect or an omission to act, or it may occur when a vulnerable person is persuaded to enter into a financial or sexual transaction to which he or she has not consented or cannot consent.*

(Department of Health, 2000a: 9)

Maltreatment of vulnerable individuals, both adults and children, can present in a variety of forms. *Table 7.1* outlines some of the key signs of which practitioners should be aware.

The term child maltreatment describes a range of ways in which individuals, often known and trusted by the child, such as a family member, family friend or a professional, harm children knowingly or by failing to act to prevent harm. Child maltreatment can be:

- Physical
- Sexual
- Due to neglect
- Emotional
- Due to fabricated/induced illness.

In many cases, children are subjected to a combination of types, such as neglect and emotional maltreatment, and this can take place in a variety of places, such as the home, school or anywhere else children spend their time. Some forms of maltreatment will be obvious, such as when an adult strikes out at a child in anger and some subtle, such as a child who appears withdrawn and tearful around a certain adult(s).

Table 7.1. Types of maltreatment in vulnerable individuals	
Types of abuse	*Examples*
Physical abuse	Slapping, pushing, kicking, misuse of medication, restraint, or inappropriate sanctions
Psychological abuse	Emotional abuse, threats of harm or abandonment, deprivation of contact, humiliation, blaming, controlling, intimidation, coercion, harassment, verbal abuse, isolation or withdrawal from services or supportive networks
Neglect and acts of omission	Ignoring medical or physical care needs, failure to provide access to appropriate health, social care or educational services, the withholding of the necessities of life, such as medication, adequate nutrition and heating
Sexual abuse	Rape and sexual assault or sexual acts to which the vulnerable adult has not consented, or could not consent or was pressured into consenting
Discriminatory abuse	Racism, sexism, or abuse based on a person's disability, other forms of harassment, slurs or similar treatment
Financial or material abuse	Theft, fraud, exploitation, pressure in connection with wills, property or inheritance or financial transactions, or the misuse or misappropriation of property, possessions or benefits

The legal framework

The legal framework is provided principally by the Children Act 1999 in England and Wales (OPSI, 1999), the Children (Scotland) Act 1995 (OPSI, 1995a) and the Children (Northern Ireland) Order 1995 (OPSI, 1995b). Each sets out the powers and responsibilities of local authorities and the means by which children can be safeguarded and their welfare promoted. In England and Wales, the updated Children Act 2004 (OPSI, 2004) places a statutory duty on key individuals and organisations, including healthcare professionals, to make arrangements to safeguard and promote children's welfare; to carry out their functions with regard to the safety and welfare of children; and to co-operate with other agencies through local Safeguarding Children Boards. In Northern Ireland there is a single Safeguarding Board and in Scotland vulnerable children remain the responsibility of Child Protection Committees. These bodies produce local procedures to guide all staff working with children and national guidance is also available for each country. Practitioners should make themselves aware of the relevant procedures.

Key definitions and duties

The legislation states that it is the duty of every local authority to safeguard and promote the welfare of children within their area who are "in need". Children are deemed to be in need if they are unlikely to achieve or maintain a reasonable standard of health or development without the provision of services; their health is likely to be significantly impaired, or further impaired, without the provision of services; or they are disabled; or, in Scotland, their parents are disabled (Department of Health, 2000b).

The types of child maltreatment are wide-ranging and can be extremely distressing to witness. The various types of child maltreatment and the signs and physical features that would lead a practitioner to suspect maltreatment are listed below. These signs and physical features should be documented and action taken for further investigation and appropriate ongoing referral, in accordance with local guidelines or practices. This list is comprehensive and is adapted from the National Collaborating Centre for Women's and Children's Health (2009) supported by the Royal College of Paediatrics and Child Health and further develops the current guidance in the National Service Framework for Children, Young People and Maternity Services for England (Department of Health, 2004a). These guidelines aim to raise awareness in professionals who are not specialist in child protection to the physical and psychological signs, symptoms and interactions that may alert healthcare professionals in identifying child maltreatment.

Sexual abuse

Sexual abuse involves someone (an adult or another young person) forcing or enticing a child or young person to take part in sexual activities, including prostitution, whether or not the child is aware of what is happening. The following physical features/signs prompt suspicion of sexual abuse:

- Persistent or recurrent genital or anal symptoms, e.g. bleeding or discharge.
- Genital, anal or perianal injury with no adequate medical explanation.
- Anal fissure—where constipation and Crohn's disease are excluded.
- Sexually transmitted infections, e.g. gonorrhoea, chlamydia, syphilis, genital herpes, hepatitis C, HIV or trichomonas infection in under 13-year-olds with no evidence of vertical transmission or blood contamination.
- Sexual intercourse with an under 13-year-old is unlawful—therefore any pregnancy in this age group is a sign of maltreatment.

Neglect

Neglect is defined as the persistent failure to meet a child's basic physical and/ or psychological needs, likely to seriously damage health or development. In pregnancy, this can happen as a result of maternal substance misuse. The following physical features/signs prompt suspicion of neglect:

- Medical advice not sought for a child, compromising his or her health and wellbeing, e.g. child suffering ongoing pain.
- Child who is persistently dirty and smelly – suggesting lack of care, particularly if seen in the morning.
- Repeated observation or reports about the home environment that is in parent's/carer's control, e.g. poor standard of hygiene affecting child's health, inadequate provision of food, living environment unsafe for a child's developmental stage.
- If a child has been abandoned, this constitutes maltreatment.

Emotional/behavioural abuse

Emotional/behavioural abuse is defined as the persistent emotional maltreatment of a child causing severe and persistent adverse effects on the child's emotional development. The following physical features/signs prompt suspicion of emotional/behavioural abuse:

- Child repeatedly scavenges, steals, hoards or hides food.
- Repeated or coercive sexualised behaviours or preoccupation in a prepubertal child, e.g. sexual talk associated with knowledge, drawing genitalia or emulating sexual activity.

Fabricated or induced illness (formerly known as Munchausen's syndrome)
In fabricated or induced illness a child's history or physical or psychological presentations, or findings of assessments, examinations or investigations leads to a discrepancy with a recognised clinical picture. The following physical features/signs prompt suspicion:

- Reported signs and symptoms only observed by, or occurring in the presence of, parent/carer.
- Inexplicably poor response to prescribed medication or treatment.
- New symptoms reported as soon as previous symptoms cease.
- Biologically unlikely history of events.
- Multiple opinions are sought from primary and secondary care providers and child continues to be presented with a range of signs and symptoms.
- Child's normal daily activities are limited, or he or she is using aids for activities more than deamed to be necessary.

The effects of child maltreatment

The effects of cruelty to children are wide-ranging and profound. They will vary according to the type of maltreatment and how long it has been endured but can include the following:

- Behavioural problems
- Educational problems
- Mental health problems
- Relationship difficulties
- Drug and alcohol problems
- Suicide or other self-harm
- In extreme cases, death.

It is worth remembering that the effects of maltreatment in childhood can be long-lasting; a homeless person suffering a mental health, alcohol or drug problem may have been a victim of child maltreatment in the past.

Many child maltreatment inquiries have revealed that a failure to act has resulted in serious injury or death. Information from practitioners in urgent care can be vital in preventing further maltreatment. Child protection comes before all other considerations, including patient confidentiality and the practitioner's relationship with a child's parents.

Managing potential child maltreatment cases

Guidance, funded by NICE and published by the National Collaborating Centre for Women's and Children's Health (2009), suggests a sequence of events to guide management of cases of possible child maltreatment. The following list outlines some suggested questions and issues to consider.

1. Listen and observe

- The key element to any consultation involving children.
- Take a few minutes (except in life-threatening presentations) to use these two senses of sight and sound to establish the situation.
- Document a good, comprehensive history from the parent/carer.
- Consider the following questions:
  - o Does the history match the injury?
  - o What is the child's general appearance or behaviour?
  - o Does the child appear just generally unwell, or does he or she seem withdrawn and frightened?
- Clearly document all this vital information in the clinical records.

2. Seek an explanation

- Attempt to seek an explanation for the injury/illness.
- Attempt to access any parent-held child developmental records (sometimes referred to as the "Red Book" – although the colour varies in each area).
- Confirm that the clinical presentation adequately explains the illness or injury.
- Try to establish (from documentation or otherwise):
  - o Early development
  - o Any illnesses and immunisation history
  - o Recent/previous hospital/emergency department or other visits
  - o GP and health visitor/family nurse details.

3. Record

- Document all the observations, examinations, actions and their outcomes. If child maltreatment is subsequently identified, these documents may form part of the clinical evidence for potential legal proceedings.
- Sign, date and time all entries in the clinical notes.
- Good documentation is particularly important in potential child maltreatment.

4. Consider, suspect or exclude maltreatment

- Consider child maltreatment if this is one possible explanation for the injury/illness or if the explanation for the alerting feature is included in

the differential diagnosis.
o   Identify the alerting physical features (as outlined previously).
o   Discuss, as a matter of priority, with senior colleagues, community paediatrician, child/adolescent mental health services or the designated professional for safeguarding children in your organisation or trust.
• Suspect child maltreatment if there is a serious level of concern about the possibility but no proof.
o   In such cases, the child should be referred to Young Persons or Children's Social Services
o   Depending on the severity of the injury/illness, the child may require direct transfer to hospital, if so, alert the emergency department.
o   Practitioners should also inform their line manager and/or the trust's appointed child protection officer, depending on local policy.
• Exclude child from maltreatment following discussions with senior colleagues or after gathering collateral evidence/information.

5. Record

• It may be necessary to gain further collateral information.
• This may not be your role, but as a paramedic or urgent care practitioner first on scene, you may be required to provide further information regarding the home situation.
• Remember the importance of the listening and observing. Note any history of other calls to the emergency service, or visits to the emergency department.

As in any consultation with a child, the importance of documenting an accurate and comprehensive history cannot be over-emphasised. This is the cornerstone of good clinical practice (Sibson and Brain, 2009). Any new information about possible maltreatment in a child must always trigger a referral back to the relevant social services department, the police or the NSPCC, as appropriate. Once again, it is important to document any continuing concerns in the child's notes.

As Einstein (Stearns, 2004) said, "The world is a dangerous place, not because of those who do evil, but because of those who look on and do nothing."

Duty

Gillick Competence
With respect to the concept of duty to care, in relation to competence, the assessment of the capacity of children (aged 16 years and under) to consent to treatment is described in terms of either Gillick Competence or the Fraser

Guidelines. Although these terms are used interchangeably, there are distinct differences (Wheeler, 2006). The legal age of consent in England, Wales and Northern Ireland is 18 years; in Scotland the Age of Legal Capacity is 16. However in all UK jurisdictions, an individual at age 16 is deemed competent to consent to medical treatment, unless there is a belief that they lack capacity.

The term Gillick Competence has been used in UK medical law since a 1983 case that established that any child (irrespective of age) has the ability to consent to his or her own medical treatment, without the need for parental knowledge or permission. This issue of competency was based on the House of Lords decision in *Gillick v West Norfolk and Wisbech Area Health Authority* (1985).

The case centred on Victoria Gillick, a mother of 10 children, who actively campaigned against this decision after her daughter received contraceptive advice without her knowledge. The term Gillick Competence tested whether prescribing contraception to a minor (under 16 years) without parental consent was illegal; the doctor was seen to be committing an offence by encouraging sex in a minor and giving treatment without consent. The term Gillick Competence refers to any form of medical treatment, not just contraception. The House of Lords considered whether the minor involved had given her consent. The court held that "parental rights" did not exist, other than to safeguard the best interests of a minor; the majority held that in "some circumstances a minor could consent to treatment" and that in these circumstances a parent had no power to veto treatment. Therefore children who are deemed "Gillick Competent" are able to prevent their parents from viewing their clinical records, unless consent is evident. However there is no rigid legal definition of Gillick competency and practitioners have the freedom to decide if a child is "Gillick Competent".

In the reality of everyday clinical practice, this can be challenging to all practitioners. Many young people look older than their chronological age and the availability of false identification further compounds this issue. Practitioners need to be aware of and up to date on these legal issues and also to be clear in terms of their own professional standards. The College of Paramedics makes no specific reference to either Gillick Competence or the Fraser Guidelines nor does the ECP Curriculum Framework document (Skills for Health, 2007) or the ECP Report *Right Skill, Right Time, Right Place* (Department of Health, 2004b). The Nursing and Midwifery Council's *Code of Conduct* recommends that practitioners gain consent prior to commencing any treatment or care (Nursing and Midwifery Council, 2008) and the Health Professions Council's *Standards for Conduct, Performance and Ethics* similarly states that practitioners are required to obtain informed consent prior to treatment, unless in an emergency (Health Professions Council, 2008).

Fraser Guidelines
The Fraser Guidelines emerged partly in response to the false belief that Victoria Gillick disliked having her name associated with the assessment of

children's capacity. Although this notion has been rejected, it is perpetuated by some national organisations (Wheeler, 2006). The Fraser Guidelines state that it is lawful to provide contraceptive advice and treatments to anyone aged 16 years and under, providing certain criteria are meet. These guidelines were initially outlined by Lord Fraser who suggested that HCPs had to be satisfied that the young person:

• Understands the practitioner's advice.
• Cannot be persuaded to inform his or her parents/guardians.
• Is likely to begin, or continue having, sexual intercourse with or without the use of contraceptives.
• Will suffer physical and/or mental health issues if he or she does not receive contraceptive treatment.
• Has it in their best interests to receive contraceptive advice or treatment with or without parental consent.

The significant difference between the Fraser Guidelines and Gillick Competence is that the former refers specifically to contraception, whereas Gillick Competence applies to any clinical treatment. While contraceptive treatment is perhaps not clinically defined nor regarded as urgent care from the professional's perspective, access to emergency contraception is a common reason for attending an emergency department and may be considered an urgent healthcare need by the individuals themselves (Kerins et al, 2004).

Duty of care and the ambulance service

Until recently there was no legal obligation for NHS ambulance services to provide pre-hospital care when the emergency services were summoned. Duty of care is not universally owed and this precedent was tested in 2000 in the Court of Appeal in the case of *Kent v Griffiths* (2000) in deciding that an unreasonably delayed response by an ambulance service to an emergency call could be considered negligent.

In general, English law does not hold the emergency service providers liable in negligence, whatever their failure, to help those in need. This reluctance is due to the distinction between what is referred to as acts and omissions. Acts are the harming of others by active carelessness, and omissions are simply failing to help. These are important distinctions that are essential to common law.

However, the *Kent v Griffiths* (2000) case challenged this assumption by questioning whether there was a duty of care owed by the ambulance service. In this case, the claimant, Mrs Kent, brought two simultaneous claims, one against her doctor and the other against the ambulance service.

In 1999, a GP made a house call to Mrs Kent, who was pregnant and suffering from a severe asthma attack. The GP made a 999 call, requesting an emergency ambulance and when the ambulance failed to arrive within a reasonable time, two further requests were made. Despite reassurances of an ambulance en route, the ambulance did not arrive until 40 minutes after the initial call. Mrs Kent suffered respiratory arrest, miscarriage and brain damage as a result of the asthma attack, all of which may have been prevented had the ambulance not been delayed. The Court of Appeal decided that the ambulance service was liable for compensation for the damage caused, which could have been prevented had they arrived on time. Lord Woolf (Department for Constitutional Affairs, 1996) was not prepared to accept the claim that the ambulance service was in a similar position to other emergency services, in that they did not have statutory functions.

The issue the court was required to consider was whether or not the ambulance service, in line with the other emergency services, such as the police, HM Coastguards and fire fighters, owed a duty of care to those relying on their services. Although Mrs Kent won in the first instance, the ambulance service appealed and it was determined that it was reasonable to foresee that the claimant would suffer further illness if the ambulance did not arrive promptly. Since the ambulance service had accepted the 999 call and were "sufficiently proximate", i.e. in the local vicinity, and an ambulance had been dispatched, a duty of care had therefore been established. The Court of Appeal held that it was reasonable to expect an ambulance service to have a duty of care to its patients and that such patients could expect a "prompt" response when "there was no good reason for delay". Interestingly the ambulance service would not have been considered negligent if an ambulance had not been dispatched, as duty of care would not have been established.

This particular case is significant as it was an exception to the general rule that a duty of care exists under certain circumstances. The ambulance service conceded that the patient's injuries were "foreseeable" and that the GP had clearly informed the ambulance service that Mrs Kent's condition was an emergency and this was accepted by the service, thereby accepting her status as a "patient" (a "patient" being a named person who was specifically requesting care). The ambulance was alerted to respond, suggesting that there were no conflicting priorities or other demands on the service at that time. To further compound matters, the ambulance service could offer no explanation as to the late arrival of the ambulance or as to why the documented times in the ambulance log book had been falsified. The fact that Mrs Kent had been accepted as a "patient" meant that a duty of care had been established.

For another example of a legal case see *Roe v Minister of Health* (1954).

Practical implications for urgent care

The majority of practitioners are probably not fully aware of the working of the aforementioned NHS Litigation Authority (NHSLA), despite the fact that there has been a four-fold increase in clinical negligence costs in the last decade. In a recent report, the NHSLA reported that in 2008/9 2522 clinical claims were closed with no compensation having been paid, but the total cost for processing these claims was £8.8 million.

The NHS Redress Bill (Department of Health, 2005a) and the NHS Redress Scheme (Department of Health, 2005b) were established to provide rapid resolution to clinical negligence claims, to set up an investigation framework, and to offer apology, compensation and any ongoing rehabilitative care. In the Making Amends report (Department of Health, 2003) the Chief Medical Officer set out plans for reform and review of the no-fault compensation scheme and concluded with his plans for the NHS Redress Scheme.

The delay in establishing this framework caused disquiet amongst many groups, particularly those expressly representing views of patients, such as the Patients Association and Action against Medical Accidents (AvMA). The Patients Association is a national charity established 50 years ago that supports patients in getting the best from healthcare and AvMA is an independent UK charity promoting improved patient safety and justice for individuals affected by medical accidents.

However, negligence claims are unusual against the ambulance service. A recent Care Quality Commission survey reviewed England's 11 ambulance services during July 2008 and revealed that of the patients who dialled 999 and received care from the ambulance service, 73% rated their care as "excellent" and a further 25% rated their care as either "good" or "very good". A total of 82% of patients reported that their care was explained in a way that they could fully understand. During 2007–2008, over 7 million calls were made to the 11 ambulance services, of which 25% were classed as Category C, which typically includes a wide range of minor, self-limiting types of injuries and illnesses. The ambulance services were highly rated in their response to these calls (Care Quality Commission, 2009a).

Complaints in urgent care

The Medical Defence Union (MDU) receives over 90 calls weekly from the public relating to various complaints regarding the health service. In keeping with the Care Quality Commission report (2009b) the MDU echoed some of the concerns highlighted by patients, 66% of which related to complaints concerning GP's clinical treatment, including delays in diagnosis, referral and treatment. One example was the delay in diagnosing meningitis, which has potentially disastrous consequences if overlooked.

Bacterial meningococcal meningitis is the most common form of meningitis, affecting 2000 individuals annually in the UK. The disease mainly affects young children, most of whom survive with prompt treatment and diagnosis.

Some individuals suffer long-term side effects, with 25% of survivors having a reduced quality of life.

The case of Macy, an 11-month-old baby, who died in 2006 from meningococcal septicaemia, highlights the speed at which the illness progresses. Macy's parents took her to the local emergency department` as they suspected she was suffering from meningitis. She was admitted to hospital, the relevant blood tests taken, but her blood results were not obtained until the morning of her death, despite being available hours earlier. There was no active system by which to inform the doctor or ward that the results were available. Compounded by the fact that the duty doctor was covering several clinical areas, Macy's blood results were made available too late to save her life.

Although Macy's case represents an in-hospital error, it does highlight the need for excellent communication procedures between healthcare practitioners and departments. Advice from the Health Protection Agency recommends that early treatment with benzylpenicillin, which registered paramedics are able to administer (JRCALC, 2006), in conjunction with rapid transfer to hospital will help to reduce fatalites in cases of meningitis (Health Protection Agency, 2006). A NICE consultation guideline document is currently available, with revised publication due late in 2010, which states that the pre-hospital management of suspected meningitis in children and young people should not include the administration of antibiotics if this delays urgent transfer to hospital (NICE, 2009), although clearly organisations will update and amend their policies individually in response to this guidance.

The MDU noted that the vast majority of complaints could usually be resolved very quickly in the local setting, with a prompt and sympathetic response and the offer of an apology. Approximately 2.5% of complaints to the MDU concerned out-of-hours services, and this was usually as the result of a breakdown of communication, such as not passing on a requested follow up visit from the GP. Again poor communication appears to be the key issue in claims regarding lack of duty of care.

Medical accidents are defined as avoidable harm that has been caused as a result of inappropriate treatment or the failure to treat. AvMA recently published the results of an investigation into the system of issuing patient safety alerts to NHS trusts in England. Their report *Adding Insult to Injury – NHS failure to implement patient safety alerts* (AvMA, 2010) makes depressing reading as it highlights the protracted length of time and failure to implement a number of patient safety alerts. In 2004 the National Patient Safety Agency (NPSA) was created as an arm's length body of the Department of Health to improve safe patient care through informing, supporting and influencing organisations and individuals working in the health sector. The NPSA has three functions, as a national reporting and learning service, a national clinical assessment service and a national research ethics service.

As part of the "core standards" set by the Department of Health, when the NPSA has evidence of a high priority safety issue, usually via its National Reporting and Learning Service, the issues are reviewed and assessed prior to setting a patient safety alert. Through consultations with various experts, the required actions with reasonable deadlines for implementation are decided. The patient safety alerts are usually the result of deaths or serious injury that have occurred on a repeated basis, and the NPSA is required to ensure that these alerts, which include a number of actions relevant to all NHS trusts, are implemented by the specific deadline. The key source of information for these alerts is obtained under the Freedom of Information Act's Central Alert System (OPSI, 2000).

Although *Table 7.2* represents only a small proportion of these alerts, perhaps what is most surprising is that they represent some fundamental aspects of patient care which one might assume would be implicit to good practice. Whilst ambulance trusts are easily identifiable in this document, it is more difficult to extrapolate from the data which trusts are acute and which primary care, thereby making it difficult to establish exactly what the data refer to.

Table 7.2. Completed Patient Safety Alerts January 2002–December 2009		
Patient Safety Alert	*% completed*	*Notes*
Being open when a patient is harmed	90	Featured 8 ambulance trusts
Early identification of failure to act on radiological imaging reports	83	
Improving infusion safety device	93	
Clean hands to help save lives	94	
Right patient, right blood	90	
Promoting safer measurement and administration of liquid medicines via oral and other enteral routes	86	
Risk of chest drain insertion	87	
Reducing errors with opioid medicines	79	
Reducing risk of overdose with midazolam in adults	82	
Risk to patient safety of not using the NHS Number as the national identifier for all patients	69	Updated alert
Adapted from Action Against Medical Accidents, 2010		

Summary

There are hundreds of thousands of encounters in the urgent and pre-hospital care setting every day in the UK and these are undertaken by expert practitioners, providing adequate and, in the majority of cases exceptional, levels of care. The cases highlighted in this chapter represent system failures, as opposed to the failure of specific individuals, although professionals have to be accountable for their own professional practice. It might appear easy to apportion blame to a specific individual, but hopefully the scenarios have demonstrated that in fact, it is the system that is at fault for allowin such practice to occur.

References

Action against Medical Accidents (AvMA) (2010) *Adding insult to injury – NHS failure to implement patient safety alerts*. Surrey: AvMA

Bichard Inquiry Report (2004). Available from: http://www.bichardinquiry. org.uk/

Bolam v Friern Hospital Management Committee (1957) 1 WLR 582

Buttress SJ, Marangon T (2008) Legal issues of extended practice: Where does the responsibility lie? *Radiography* **14**: 33–8

Care Quality Commission (2009a) *Ambulance services are rated highly in their response to non-urgent calls*. London: CQC

Care Quality Commission (2009b) *NHS may fail to spot patient safety concerns unless it improves monitoring of out-of-hours GP services*. London: CQC

Cawson P (2002) *Child maltreatment in the family: The experience of a national sample of young people*. London: NSPCC

Cooke MW, Wilson S, Perason S (2002) The effect of a separate stream for minor injuries on accident and emergency waiting times. *Emergency Medicine Journal* **19**(1): 28–30

Cooper MA, Lindsay GM, Kinn S, Swann IJ (2002) Evaluating Emergency Nurse Practitioner services. A randomized controlled trial. *Journal of Advanced Nursing* **40**(6): 721–30

Currie J, Crouch R (2007) How far is too far? Exploring the perceptions of the professions on their current and future roles in emergency care. *Emergency Medicine Journal* **25**(6): 335–9

Department for Constitutional Affairs (1996) *Access to Justice. Final Report by the Right Honourable the Lord Woolf, Master of the Rolls. Final Report to the Lord Chancellor on the civil justice system in England and Wales*. London: HMSO

Department of Health (1996) *Childhood matters. Report of the National Commission of Inquiry into the Prevention of Child Abuse*. Vol. 2. London: HMSO

Department of Health (2000a) *No secrets. Guidance on developing and implementing multi agency policies and procedures to protect vulnerable adults from maltreatment*. London: TSO

Department of Health (2000b) *Framework for the assessment of children in need and their families*. London: HMSO

Department of Health (2000c) *The NHS Plan: A Plan for Investment, a Plan for Reform*. London: HMSO

Department of Health (2003) *Making amends: A consultation paper setting out proposals for reforming the approach to clinical negligence in the NHS*. London: HMSO

Department of Health (2004a) *National Service Framework for Children, Young People and Maternity Services*. London: HMSO

Department of Health (2004b) *The ECP Report: Right Skills, Right Time, Right Place*. London: HMSO

Department of Health (2005a) *NHS Redress Bill*. London: TSO

Department of Health (2005b) *NHS Redress Scheme*. London: TSO.

Department of Health (2006) *Modernising nursing careers – Setting the direction*. London: HMSO

Department of Health (2009) *The European Working Time Directive for trainee doctors – Implementation update*. London: HMSO

Dobbie AE, Cooke MW (2008) A descriptive review and discussion of litigation claims against ambulance services. *Emergency Medicine Journal* 25(7): 455–8

Dowling S, Martin R, Skidmore P, Doyal L, Cameron A , Lloyd S (1996) Nurses taking on junior doctors' work: A confusion of accountability. *British Medical Journal* **312**: 1211–14

Ezra DG, Mellington F, Cugnoni H, Westcott M (2005) Reliability of ophthalmic accident and emergency referrals: A new role for the emergency nurse practitioner? *Emergency Medicine Journal* **22**(9): 696–9

Gillick v West Norfolk and Wisbech Area Health Authority [1985] 3 All ER 402 (HL)

Griffith R, Tengnah C (2009) Understanding the Safeguarding Vulnerable Groups Act 2006. *British Journal of Community Nursing* **14**(7): 309–13

Health Professions Council (2008) *Standards of Conduct, Performance and Ethics*. London: HPC

Health Protection Agency (2006) *Guidance for public health manage-*

ment of meningococcal disease in the UK. Health Protection Agency Meningococcus Forum (Updated August 2006)

JRCALC (Joint Royal Colleges Ambulance Liaison Committee) (2006) *Benzylpenicillin (Penicillin G)*. Warwick: JRCALC

Kaye P, Taylor C, Barley K, Powell-Chandler A (2009) An emergency department intervention to protect an overlooked group of children at risk of significant harm. *Emergency Medicine Journal* **26**(6): 415–17

Kent v Griffiths [2000] 2 All ER 474

Kerins M, Maguire E, Fahey DK, Glucksman E (2004) Emergency contraception. Has over the counter availability reduced attendances at emergency departments? *Emergency Medicine Journal* **21**(1): 67–8

Laming H (2003) *The Victoria Climbié Inquiry Report*. London. HMSO

National Audit Office (2006) *The provision of out-of-hours care in England*. London: TSO

National Collaborating Centre for Women's and Children's Health (2009) *When to suspect child maltreatment*. London: RCOG Press

National Health Service Litigation Authority (2009/10) *NHSLA risk management standards for acute trusts, primary care rrusts and independent sector providers of NHS care*. London: NHSLA

National Health Service Litigation Authority (2010/11) *NHSLA risk management standards for ambulance trusts*. London: NHSLA

NICE (National Institute for Health and Clinical Excellence) (2009) *Draft Consultation: Bacterial meningitis and meningococcal septicaemia: Management of bacterial meningitis and meningococcal septicaemia in children and young people younger than 16 years in primary and secondary care*. London: NICE

NSPCC (2008) *Child protection register statistics – Northern Ireland 2004–2008*. London: NSPCC

NSPCC (2009) *Child protection register statistics - Wales 2005–2009*. London: NSPCC

Nursing and Midwifery Council (2008) *Code. Standards of conduct, performance and ethics for nurses and midwives*. London: NMC

Ofsted (2008) *Annual Report of Her Majesty's Chief Inspector of Education, Children's Services and Skills 2007/08*. London: The Stationary Office

OPSI (Office of Public Sector Information) (1995a) *Children (Scotland) Act 1995*. London: OPSI.

OPSI (Office of Public Sector Information) (1995b) *Children (Northern Ireland) Order 1995*. London: OPSI

OPSI (Office of Public Sector Information) (1999) *Protection of Children Act 1999*. London: OPSI

OPSI (Office of Public Sector Information) (2000) *Freedom of Information Act 2000*. London: OPSI

OPSI (Office of Public Sector Information) (2004) *Children Act 2004*. London: OPSI

OPSI (Office of Public Sector Information) (2006) *Safeguarding Vulnerable Adults Act 2006*. London: OPSI

Richards DA, Meakins J, Godfrey L, Tawfik J, Dutton E (2004) Survey of the impact of nurse telephone triage in general practitioner activity. *British Journal of General Practice* **54**(500): 207–10

Roe v Minister of Health (1954) 2 All ER 131

Scottish Executive (1999) *Protecting Children: A Shared Responsibility*. Edinburgh: Scottish Executive

Sibson L, Brain L (2009) Safeguarding children: Role of health professionals. *Journal of Paramedic Practice* **1**(12): 493–500

Sidebotham P, Biu T, Goldsworthy L (2007) Child protection procedures in emergency departments. *Emergency Medicine Journal* **24**(12): 831–5

Skills for Health (2006) *Measuring the benefits of the emergency care practitioner*. Bristol: Skills for Health

Skills for Health (2007) *The competence and curriculum framework for the emergency care practitioner*. Bristol: Skills for Health

Stearns M (2004) *Conscious Courage: Turning Everyday Challenges Into Opportunities*. Florida: Enrichment Books

Wheeler R (2006) Editorial: Gillick or Fraser? A plea for consistency over competence in children. *British Medical Journal* **332**(7541): 807

Williams K (2007) Litigation against English NHS Ambulance Service and the Rule in *Kent v. Griffiths*. In *Medical Law Review*. Oxford: Oxford University Press

Woodman J, Pitt M, Wentz R, Taylor B, Hodes D, Gilbert RE (2008) Performance of screening tests for child physical abuse in accident and emergency departments. *Health Technology Assessment* **12**(33):xi–xiii; 1–95

CHAPTER 8

Ethical issues

This chapter on ethical issues is underpinned by the four key ethical principles of autonomy, nonmaleficence, beneficence, and justice. These principles are generic, and to some extent overlap with some of the legal principles discussed in *Chapter 7*. The role of ethics is to seek a beneficial balance between the activities of an individual and their effect on society as a whole. All four ethical principles underpin healthcare practice and also represent the fundamental principles in research. These four "pillars" are therefore essential and each will be discussed in relation to urgent care (see *Figure 8.1*).

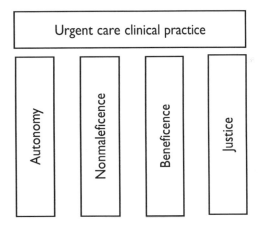

Figure 8.1. The four pillars of ethical principles.

Autonomy

Autonomy originated from Ancient Greece meaning "*auto*" or self and "*nomos*" or law, or "one who gives oneself law". Autonomy essentially refers to the capacity of a rational individual to make an informed, un-coerced decision. The concept of autonomy in healthcare largely works to ensure that any unjustified paternalism is kept to a minimum. Therefore autonomy is viewed as the right of the patient to make a decision, as long as the patient is able to understand and appreciate his or her condition, prognosis and the risks and benefits of any proposed treatment to arrive at a decision to relay to the practitioner (Swindell, 2009).

Autonomy from a philosophical perspective is based on essentially having responsibility for one's action. The German philosopher Immanuel Kant (1724–1804) developed one of the more common philosophical theories relating to autonomy. Often referred to as Kantianism, Kant's philosophical principles related to the utilitarian or deontological principles of ethics. Kant's philosophical stance was "Do unto others as you would have done unto you". Kant's principle was that an act is right if, and only if, it conforms to an overriding moral obligation and is wrong if it violates a moral duty or principle. Deontological ethics holds that some acts are morally wrong; such as lying or breaking a promise.

Similarly, the English philosopher John Stuart Mill (1806–1873) developed the "greatest happiness" principle. This was based on the utilitarian principle of the "greatest happiness for the greatest number of people", but within reason. Utilitarianism aims to answer the question of what one ought to do.

In medicine, respect for the autonomy of the patient is one of the fundamental principles of healthcare. This has been shaped and developed over 50 years following the Nuremberg trials, which examined the horrific medical experiments that were performed in the concentration camps during World War II. The Nuremberg trials were a series of military tribunals that set out to investigate, and eventually prosecute, a number of prominent political and military leaders. This subsequently had a substantial impact on the development of international criminal law and these incidents also promoted the need for safeguards in medical research. The term "informed consent" was adopted after the trials, although it did not come into standard use until the 1970s.

The Nuremberg Code

The resulting Nuremberg Code led to the development of the Medical Ethics Committee of the World Medical Association in the 1950s. It proposed an ethical policy for research and the subsequent proposals are perhaps better known as the Declaration of Helsinki (World Medical Association, 1964). These proposals represented a detailed framework for research, including the basic principles for clinical and non-clinical therapeutic trials. Subsequent revisions of the Declaration include the protection of minors in research, and although there are many updated versions, the European Commission refers to the fourth version published in 1996.

Some critics suggest that the principle of autonomy overrides all other ethical principles, although this is not a view held by all (Beauchamp and Childress, 2009). An autonomous individual is defined as one who acts freely, in accordance with a self-chosen plan. By contrast, individuals with decreased autonomy are in some way controlled by others and incapable of acting on the basis of their own plans. Such individuals include those with severe learning difficulties or mental illness. Incapacity is considered present if an individual is unable to understand and intelligently act upon consent information using a rational process of mental status. Autonomy is a general indicator of health and since many illnesses cause some degree of a loss of autonomy it can be viewed as a gauge of an individual's well-being.

Informed consent

Informed consent is a legal term used to indicate that an individual has provided consent that meets some minimal agreed standard. In order to provide informed consent, individuals need to be in possession of all the facts at the time the consent is provided. Failure to gain informed consent prior to a procedure can result in the practitioner being liable for battery. Exceptions to gaining informed consent include severe mental illness and learning difficulties, intoxication, sleep deprivation and coma. The law of informed consent legally expresses the ethical principle of autonomy and respect for autonomy. Historically, informed consent was not routinely required in healthcare, but related almost exclusively to research. The core principle of autonomy recognises the right of an individual to self-determination, with its central premise being that of informed consent and shared decision-making.

In an emergency, as is frequently the case in urgent care, consent is presumed, particularly if the patient is unconscious, in severe pain or has a life-threatening illness or injury (Health Professions Council, 2008; College of Paramedics/British Paramedics Association, 2008). Since consent is largely implied in emergency cases, it tends to become assumed and is, perhaps, all to often, overlooked.

For a legal case example, see: *Salgo v Leland Stanford Jr. University* (1957)
Informed consent used in court of law for the first time

Beauchamp and Childress (2009) outlined seven elements of informed consent. Their listing is based upon on a range of literature from the legal, philosophical, medical and regulatory fields and is outlined in *Table 8.1*.

In applying the majority of Beauchamp and Childress' elements of informed consent, it is worth considering a hypothetical but perhaps, to some readers, unfortunately all too familiar situation. *Box 8.1* outlines a patient consultation that demonstrates the problems of gaining informed consent.

It should be remembered that even in an emergency situation, practitioners should still attempt to gain consent as far as possible. Patients also have the right to refuse treatment and this must be respected and documented. However patients should be made fully aware of the risks of refusing any treatment, particularly if, as a paramedic, you think there would be a "significant or immediate risk to life" (Health Professions Council, 2008: 12).

Table 8.1. Seven elements of informed consent	
Elements	*Explanation*
Threshold (or pre-requites)	
1. Competence	To understand the information regarding the proposed care*
2. Voluntariness	To decide to undertake proposed care
Information elements	
3. Disclosure	Awareness of information related to proposed care
4. Recommendation	Recomending proposed plan of care
5. Understanding	Understanding of Disclosure and Recommendation (3 and 4)
Consent elements	
6. Decision (for or against plan of care)	In favour/opposed to proposed care
7. Authorisation (for or against plan of care)	Consent/refusal for proposed care
* Proposed care in this context refers to any form of procedure/treatment that a practitioner may carry out on a patient	
	Adapted from Beauchamp and Childress (2009)

Box 8.1. Scenario: Joe

A paramedic practitioner is called to attend Joe, a male patient in his late 30s who has been found semi-conscious in the street. Joe is complaining of headaches and nausea and, on initial assessment, appears to have sustained head trauma with some lacerations and bruising to his occipital area. In addition, Joe smells strongly of alcohol and appears unkempt and malnourished. Joe has significant nicotine staining on his fingers and numerous needle marks on his arms and feet, with evidence of infection to a number of these sites. On further examination, it is clear that his head wounds require hospital treatment, and his semi-conscious state and probable drug and alcohol use would also require some further assessment and treatment.

Initially Joe refuses to attend the emergency department, but after some gentle persuasion on the part of the practitioner, he concedes to be transferred to hospital for treatment of his head wounds. Once in the ambulance, he admits to having been assaulted on the previous evening and cannot recall events since this time, suggesting a period of unconsciousness.

Once Joe has been admitted to the emergency department, the practitioner makes his concerns known to the senior doctor on call. However, Joe has now retracted his story of being assaulted as he does not wish to have any contact with the police.

Competence

According to Beauchamp and Childress' first element, the practitioner would need to ensure that the patient was competent to give an informed consent. This immediately raises the issue that in an unconscious patient, assessment of competence is clearly challenging. There is a variety of tests available to assess the range or level of competence to determine if a patient possesses time and space orientation, including the Glasgow Coma Scale. In urgent care, such assessments need to be undertaken promptly.

Voluntariness

Voluntariness is the patient's right to make a healthcare choice that is free from any influence, a pre-requisite to informed consent. In Joe's case, although it took some gentle persuasion on the part of the practitioner to attend the emergency department, he did eventually consent to be transferred to hospital for treatment. Although Joe appeared to have attended without any apparent coercion, the practitioner should be mindful that his attendance does not necessarily mean the practitioner should desist from encouraging patients to accept their advice. The patient still has the right to accept or reject that advice. It is important that the practitioner ensures that Joe's actions are not controlled by others (Etchells, 1996).

Disclosure and recommendation

Disclosure is vital in the informed decision making process and without the ability of the urgent care professional to be an "agent of disclosure", patients will have insufficient information on which to base their decisions. The general rule is that professionals are obliged to provide key information, including any facts that aid the patient's decision either to consent or to refuse treatment/intervention, and the information has to be material and recommended by the professional. In relation to urgent care, there are a number of relevant Acts which require practitioners to disclose information and these are outlined in *Table 8.2*. Patients often view the disclosure of information as less important than that of the practitioner's recommendation of the plan of action (Beauchamp and Childress, 2009).

For a legal case example, see: *Rogers v Whitaker* (1992)
Case focusing on issues of disclosure

Understanding

Patients should have an understanding of the information regarding their proposed care and treatment. Potential limitations to a patient's understanding in the consent process arise if patients are anxious, distressed or in pain. Other elements of language and/or cultural barriers, and the presence of mental health issues or learning difficulties hamper understanding. Whilst there is no

Table 8.2. Laws that require disclosure	
Statute	*Requirement*
• Public Health (Control of Disease) Act 1984 (OPSI, 1984)	Requires the reporting of notifiable diseases such as chlolera, plague and relapsing fever
• Road Traffic Act 1998 (OPSI, 1998a)	Requires notification to the police of any individual suspected to be guilty of contravention of this Act
• Terrorism Act 2000 (OPSI, 2000b)	Requires the reporting of information relating to the commision of acts of terrorism contrary to the Act
• Public Health (Infectious Diseases) Regulations 1998 (OPSI, 1998b) • Public Health etc. (Scotland) Act 2008 (OPSI, 2008) • Public Health Act (Northern Ireland) 1967 (OPSI, 1967)	Require the medical practitioner to provide patient's name, address, sex, date of birth, organism and transmission (if known) and NHS identifier for diseases including acquired immune deficiency syndrome, malaria, measles, meningitis, scarlet fever, etc.
	Adapted from Peate and Potterton (2009)

consensus on the nature of understanding per se, as long as patients have a grasp of the pertinent details, patients are adequately informed. The essential facts are the vital facts that might be decisive enough for a decision to be made. Patients should understand the diagnosis, prognosis, nature and purpose of interventions, and the alternatives, risks and benefits. The use of lay language is important as medical terms can lead to confusion. Ensuring that patients are fully informed of all interventions can be challenging; ensuring that they are adequately informed may be more achievable. In addition, providing too much information can also inhibit the decision making process and information overload can result in patients being unable to meaningfully organise and absorb information.

Decision

Decisions can include the acceptance or refusal of treatment. Giving informed consent for a clinical examination is relevant in urgent care since the vast majority of presenting patients have undifferentiated problems with often limited or no access to existing clinical records. Patients may also be unable to consent because of altered consciousness, due to intoxication or a coma, as highlighted in Joe's case. Generally speaking, "consent" or "true consent" is a due process under which the practitioner explains to the patient the nature of the treatment s/he intends to provide. Practitioners should provide material information as would be provided by their peers in similar circumstances, although they may withhold such information if it is felt to be harmful to the patient to know. This is sometimes referred to as therapeutic privilege. The patient would then offer agreement to treatment – so the profession decides on what the patient needs to know.

Authorisation

Authorisation of the chosen plan can then be provided, often verbally or, in the case of the urgent or emergency situation, concurrently with life-saving treatment.

In emergency situations, informed consent may not be necessary or possible, as providing urgent pre-hospital care is considered the foremost requirement (Foëx, 2001). For example, seriously injured patients requiring treatment that is prohibited by their religious or ethical beliefs is often challenging. Dimond (1993) cites the case of *Malette v Shulman* (1991) in Canada where Mrs Malette, a 57-year-old woman, was seriously injured in a car accident and was transferred to hospital in an unconscious state. It was discovered that she was a Jehovah's Witness and was carrying instructions stating no blood transfusions were to be administered under any circumstances. The doctor was informed but administered a blood transfusion, deciding it was clinically necessary. The patient made a good recovery but sued the doctor for negligence, assault, battery and religious discrimination. The judge only accepted the plea to battery, having concluded that the instructions restricted the doctor's right to administer blood and awarded Mrs Malette damages.

Regulatory guidance on informed consent in urgent care

As we have seen, obtaining informed consent in the urgent care setting presents specific challenges. The vast majority of legal advice refers to the medical profession – with only some specific guidance to allied health professionals. The Nursing and Midwifery Council (NMC) refers specifically to consent in relation to the covert administration of medications (NMC, 2008a).

With the respect to professional standards, the NMC's Code of Conduct (2008b) states that nurses should respect patients' rights to confidentiality, ensuring that patients are informed about how and why information is shared by those who will be providing their care. The disclosure of information is only recommended when, as a practitioner, you believe someone may be at risk of harm, in line with the law of the country in which you are practising. In an emergency, the NMC Code of Conduct further states that nurses must be able to demonstrate that they have acted in someone's best interests if they have provided care in an "emergency". The Standards of Proficiency for Paramedics (Health Professions Council, 2007) states that paramedics, as part of their professional autonomy and accountability, must understand the importance of, and be able to maintain, confidentiality, and obtain informed consent

The Joint Royal Colleges Ambulance Liaison Committee (JRCALC)

Clinical Guidelines (2006b) are perhaps more helpful, suggesting the following three prompt questions:

*   *Does the patient have the capacity to consent?* Ensure that the patient comprehends and retains the information and uses it to make a decision.
*   *Is the consent given voluntarily?* Consent is only valid if it is freely given with no pressure or influence to accept or refuse treatment.
*   *Has the patient received sufficient information?* Ensure the patient understands the nature and purpose of a treatment and the potential consequences of consenting to, or refusal of, consent. Failure to provide all relevant information may render the paramedic liable to an action for negligence.

From a regulatory perspective, the Quality Assurance Agency (QAA) subject benchmark statement for paramedics outlines that "informed consent" should be achieved, where appropriate, with patients/clients (QAA, 2004: 13).

Similarly, the QAA subject benchmark statements for nurses states that practitioners need to "understand the legal and ethical responsibilities of professional practice" (QAA, 2001: 2). The College of Paramedics/British Paramedic Association refers to informed consent in its curriculum guidance and recommends the teaching of ethics and law for practice, which should address ethical and legal frameworks, such as the principles of autonomy, beneficence, maleficence and non-maleficence. However, no further guidance is provided on the nature of the sessions (College of Paramedics/British Paramedic Association, 2008). The College of Paramedics/British Paramedic Association also recommend that "paramedics have an understanding of the ethical and legal contexts in which they operate" (College of Paramedics/ British Paramedic Association, 2008: 50).

Unfortunately none of the above organisations defines either what specifically constitutes an "emergency" or "informed consent" although local trust policies may provide some further guidance. One could argue that all calls to the ambulance service are an emergency, at least from the patient's perspective. Perhaps an assumption is made therefore, that all calls and subsequent cases constitute an emergency until established otherwise?

To undertake any treatment without informed consent, whilst this is poorly defined for paramedics and nurses, legally constitutes battery. Battery is essentially physical assault, for example, hitting or touching an individual without permission, with ill intent. This therefore constitutes a crime and is dealt with under criminal law. In addition, "trespass" implies negligence; an example being that a doctor owed a duty of care to a patient by way of providing sufficient information before a procedure and, having failed to do so, if the patient is harmed, the patient can then sue the doctor for negligence.

To respect autonomy is to acknowledge the right of individuals to hold views, to make choices and to take action based on their personal values and beliefs. As such, this respect for autonomy involves what Beauchamp and Childress (2009) refer to as action and not merely a respectful attitude. This centres on the non-interference into another's personal affairs. The concept of respect, in this context, involves the acknowledgement of the value of the decision-making right of individuals by enabling them to act autonomously. Disrespect for autonomy, in the other hand, involves those actions and attitudes that ignore, demean, insult or are inattentive to other's rights to autonomy.

Criminally inflicted injuries

One particular area of clinical care that is specifically challenging is the issue of consent in injuries resulting from violent criminal activity – particularly as a result of knife and gun crime. The number of criminally inflicted injuries in emergency department patients is, despite media reports to the contrary, remaining constant. In the previous decade, knife crime accounted for approximately 7% of all violent incidents. Whilst the frequency of knife crime remains constant, the severity of the associated injury appears to have increased (Hughes, 2009). The General Medical Council (GMC) recently published guidelines for doctors outlining their responsibility for reporting knife crime. In the case of criminally inflicted injuries, the new GMC guidance recommends that the police are contacted, since they remain responsible for assessing the risk posed to hospital staff, and should therefore be informed of any violent, deliberate knife wounds. If patients refuse to disclose personal information or are unable to provide consent they can be overruled if health professionals believe there are grounds that justify information disclosure in the interest of public safety. Of course the patient's consent to disclosure should be sought whenever possible (GMC, 2009).

Similarly, the management of gunshot injuries in the urgent care setting has also been addressed in recent GMC guidance. The recommendations advise that emergency departments should report all gunshot injuries to the police (GMC, 2009). However Frampton (2005) questions whether gun crime, above other types of violent crime, warrants this breach of patient confidentiality. The GMC states, "If a patient's refusal to consent to disclosure leaves others exposed to a risk so serious that it outweighs the patient's and the public interest in maintaining confidentiality, you should disclose information promptly to an appropriate person or authority." (GMC, 2009:1).

Informed consent and children

In relation to children, in Europe the rights granted to children under the European Convention in Human Rights (Council of Europe, 1950) and the Human Rights Act (1998) in the UK are not sacrosanct and are therefore not legal rights. The Medical Protection Society (2008) states that in an emergency situation, if a person with parental responsibility is unavailable, the doctor has to consider the child's best interests and act appropriately. Treatment should be limited to that which is reasonably required to manage the specific emergency, and all decisions taken should be documented, with the supporting rationale.

Data protection

Documentation is fundamental in patient care, not least from the legal and ethical perspectives. Following on from the theme of informed consent, data protection is explored in the context of the ethical principle of autonomy. In the UK, the Data Protection Act (OPSI, 1998c) affords individuals the right to know what information is held about them whilst providing a framework to ensure that the information is handled correctly. The Data Protection Act works in two ways. First, all healthcare professionals processing personal patient information must comply with the eight data protection principles listed in *Table 8.3*.

Second, the Act provides individuals with important rights, including access to electronic and paper records containing any personal information held about them. The Act defines personal data as information relating to a living individual, who could potentially be identified from that data or other information, which could come into the possession of the data controller (a data controller is an individual who determines the purposes and manner in which any personal data about an individual is to be processed). Data, in this respect, is defined as information which is either processed or recorded.

The right for individuals to review their health records was introduced by the Access to Health Records Act (OPSI, 1988). In 2000, the Data Protection Act partly replaced the Access to Health Records Act, which did not cover access to manual records held before 24th October 1998 and which, unlike the Data Protection Act, concerns access to records of deceased patients. Exemptions to the Access to Health Records Act refers to medical practitioners

Table 8.3. Eight principles of the Data Protection Act 1998	
Principle 1	Data should be fairly and lawfully processed
Principle 2	Data should be processed for limited purposes
Principle 3	Data should be adequate, relevant and not excessive
Principle 4	Data should be accurate and up to date
Principle 5	Data should not be kept for longer than is necessary
Principle 6	Data should be processed in line with your rights
Principle 7	Data should be secure
Principle 8	Data should not be transferred to other countries without adequate protection

only in that they are not obliged to provide individual access to any part of a medical report "whose disclosure, in the opinion of the practitioner, would be likely to cause serious harm to the physical or mental health of the patients or others" (OPSI, 1988: 4; 2000a). The medical practitioner is also obliged not to disclose any part of a medical report that would reveal the identity of another person, or information from another individual, unless the individual concerned has consented or the person is a health professional involved in the patient's care.

The Caldicott Report

With this is mind, the Caldicott Committee, chaired by Dame Fiona Caldicott and commissioned by the Department of Health, set out to review all patient-identifiable information that passes from NHS to non-NHS organisations for the purposes of care, research or that which is a statutory requirement in relation to security and confidentiality. The purpose of the Committee was to ensure that only the minimum patient-identifiable information was transferred, and that it was for justified purposes and with minimal breaches in confidentiality. The Committee made a number of recommendations and identified six key principles, which became known as the Caldicott Guidelines (Department of Health, 1997). Following the publication of the Caldicott Guidelines, NHS organisations were obliged to appoint Caldicott guardians who were to ensure that the guidelines were appropriately implemented. These guardians were senior health professionals, usually in a senior management position, who had the ability to influence policy and strategy within the organisation. The six key principles of the Caldicott Guidelines are:

- *Justify the purpose(s)*: Every proposed use or transfer of patient-identifiable information within or from an organisation should be clearly defined and scrutinised. An appropriate guardian should regularly review any continuing use of such information.
- *Do not use patient-identifiable information unless it is absolutely necessary*: Patient-identifiable information items should not be included unless it is essential for the specified purpose(s) of that flow. The need for patients to be identified should be considered at each stage of satisfying the purpose(s).
- *Use the minimum necessary patient-identifiable information*: Where use of such information is considered essential, the inclusion of each individual item of information should be considered and justified so that the minimum amount of necessary information for a given function to be carried out is transferred or accessed.
- *Access to patient-identifiable information should be on a strict need to know basis*: Only those individuals who need access to such information should have access to it, and they should only have access to the items

that they need to see. This may mean introducing access controls or splitting information flows where one information flow is used for several purposes.

- *Everyone with access to patient-identifiable information should be aware of his or her responsibilities*: Action should be taken to ensure that those handling patient-identifiable information – both clinical and non-clinical staff – are made fully aware of their responsibilities and obligations to respect patient confidentiality.
- *Understand and comply with the law*: Every use of patient-identifiable information must be lawful. Someone in each organisation handling patient information should be responsible for ensuring that the organisation complies with legal requirements.

The basic premise of the Caldicott Report was that patient information was deemed to be confidential to the patient and should not be disclosed without the patient's express consent, unless justified for a lawful purpose. In urgent care, where individuals may be unable to provide consent, the decision would be made on the patient's behalf by those responsible for providing care, taking into account the views of patient, relatives or carers, with the individual's best interests being paramount. Where practicable, advice should be sought from the nominated senior professional and the reasons for the final decision should be clearly documented.

For a legal case example, see: *W v Egdell* (1990)
Case focusing on issue of disclosure (Harbour, 1998)

The later document on confidentiality published by the Department of Health (2003b) defined patient-identifiable information as that which contained the following: patient's name, address, postcode, date of birth, photographs, video or audio tapes or any other images of the patient, NHS number, local patient-identifiable codes and any other data that would identify a patient either directly or indirectly. This document also outlined guidance on the best practice for record keeping and maintaining confidentiality of patient information.

Data protection issues in clinical practice

A paper by Ayatollahi et al (2009) explored the issues in their emergency department study, demonstrating that in the majority of patients, access to their medical history was actually not required, since most presenting conditions were relatively isolated, for example fractures or abrasions as the result of falls. However in a minority of patients, access to their clinical records was required, for example in patients with cardiac conditions or previous emergency department attendances. Accessing records from other hospitals or organisations potentially created an increased risk of a confidentiality breach, since the notes are required to be handled by a number of non-clinical individuals.

However, accessing primary care records was considered vital, particularly in relation to any known allergies and immunisation status. Similarly, access to any social information was important, particularly in the management of older patients where this social information can influence decisions in patient admission. The Ayatollahi et al study revealed that accessing primary care and social service information was challenging. GPs were frequently unavailable, particularly out of hours, to provide access to notes, and social services are reluctant to share information due to confidentiality issues. The authors concluded that whilst electronic records were of value with regard to accessing the correct information, the practitioner's requirements should be considered in addition to addressing patient confidentiality issues.

There is more published guidance relating to confidentiality, the majority of which is based on generic principles but, with common sense, this is adaptable to paramedic and nursing practice. The availability of specific and detailed guidance, specifically for the urgent and pre-hospital care setting will undoubtedly be available in the future.

For a legal case example, see: *D v NSPCC* (1978)
Alleged child maltreatment focusing on public interest immunity

Nonmaleficence

Nonmaleficence is derived from the Latin phrase "*primum non* (or *nil) nocere*" implying the doctrine "first, do no harm" or "above all, do no harm". Non-maleficence is a fundamental ethical principle, pertinent to urgent healthcare, reminding practitioners that good intentions may have unwanted consequences or "sometimes the cure is worse than the ill".

Whilst the term is frequently used, its origins are actually less clear. The Hippocratic Oath, well known to doctors, includes the promise "to abstain from doing harm". However it would appear that this is not actually taken from the teaching of Hippocrates, as most people assume. Further investigation by Smith (2005) suggested the English physician Thomas Sydenham (1642–1689) often referred to as the "English Hippocrates", was the source:

> *Lest it should be objected that our opinions are new-fangled, and therefore unworthy of credence, we crouch under the cloak of Sydenham, and say, that our motto is none other that a translation of his Latin aphorism respecting a physician's duties, viz.:"Primum est ut non nocere"*

Smith (2005: 372)

From a nursing perspective, Florence Nightingale in her 1863 text, *Notes on Hospitals*, said:

179

It may seem a strange principle to enunciate as the very first requirement in a hospital that it should do the sick no harm.

Nightingale (1863)

Loefler argues that the Hippocratic Oath does not of course take into account some of the elements of modern medicine, such as access to abortion and assisted suicide, and many of today's therapeutic interventions inevitably carry some degree of risk of harm to the patient (Loefler, 2002).

While the concept of doing no harm is indeed laudable, and one practitioners strive to achieve, it in fact only represents half of the story. Merely avoiding harm does not meet with the challenges of improving patients' health, alleviating suffering and curing disease. Smith (2005) argued that the maxim of "do no harm" is a directive not a proverb and proverbs have, by definition, different meanings on different levels and can therefore be applied to a variety of situations.

Nonmaleficence is perhaps therefore better simply defined as "do no harm" and requires practitioners not to provide ineffective or purposefully harmful treatment to their patients. However this is not a particularly useful guide, since many beneficial treatments carry potentially serious side effects. However the important ethical principle here is that the benefit of any such treatment outweighs any potential burden. The principle of nonmaleficence is therefore most useful when balanced against maleficence.

Practitioners should not provide ineffective treatments that offer little hope of bringing benefit to patients. Additionally, practitioners should not do anything that purposively harms patients, and this action should be balanced against proportional benefits. As many interventions, such as medications, procedures and investigations, often bring some element of harm to patients, the principle of nonmaleficence therefore provides little guidance.

Examples of nonmaleficence include stopping a medication that has been shown to be harmful or refusing to provide a treatment that is proven ineffective.

The distinction should be made between "doing no harm" through an act of omission, and acts of harm themselves. The medical profession tends to adopt a utilitarian approach – that of the greatest good being accomplished through public action. The obligations of not harming others are quite distinct from omission (e.g. not administering penicillin to a patient with a known penicillin allergy) and the obligation to help others (e.g. providing patients with crutches to prevent further damage to an injured joint). Taking this further, in public health research for example, a vaccination programme involves asking individuals to participate in studies involving vaccines and screening. In the theory of utilitarian ethics, this would be seen to result in more good than harm for the population as a whole. But the simple differentiation between nonmaleficence and beneficence is perhaps not so straightforward.

Frankena (1973) cited in Beauchamp and Childress (2009) divided the principle of beneficence into four general obligations, which included:

- One should not to inflict evil or harm.
- One should prevent evil or harm.
- One should remove evil or harm.
- One should do or promote good.

The first obligation of not inflicting evil or harm, Beauchamp and Childress (2009) identified as nonmaleficence, whilst the remaining three refer to beneficence. Beauchamp and Childress noted that combining both ethical concepts, as many authors have a tendency to do, actually obscures some of the important aspects of each. An obligation not to harm others (preventing killing and disablement) and an obligation to help others (promoting health and providing various benefits) are distinctly different. The obligation not to harm an individual tends to be more stringent that the obligation to assist them.

One example is causing very minor localised skin irritation following administration of a potentially life-saving vaccine to a child, in this instance the obligation of beneficence (promoting health) outweighs that of nonmaleficence (not causing harm). The risk of harm, usually very small, is far outweighed by the benefits to society.

> For a legal case example, see: *Maynard v West Midlands Regional Health Authority* (1985)
> Case where Judge's preference for one body of expert opinion over another is not sufficient to establish negligence (Norrie, 1985)

The measles, mumps and rubella (MMR) vaccine debate

The MMR vaccine scandal followed the now infamous article published in *The Lancet* by Dr Andrew Wakefield and his colleagues. The original article (Wakefield et al, 1998), which included 11 other authors (10 of whom subsequently withdrew their support), was launched at a press conference in London. It lead to many years of clinical debate and parental confusion as to the efficacy and side effects of the MMR vaccine offered to children in early childhood. Wakefield and his colleagues initially claimed that a new syndrome of bowel disease and autism appeared in a number of children following administration of the combined MMR vaccine. The article reported on a study of 12 children, diagnosed with a spectrum of autism disorders, allegedly linked to the MMR vaccine. It stated that although there was no casual connection proven, it was recommended that the measles, mumps and rubella components of the vaccine be separated by a year.

Subsequent studies have been unable to reproduce Wakefield's findings (Black et al, 2002) and the Department of Health would not support the single vaccine, since there was no evidence base, it would be costly and inconvenient, and would cause greater distress to children, not least in relation to the issue of compliance. The original article was retracted in 2001 and Dr Wakefield was found guilty of serious professional misconduct in May 2010 (General Medical Council, 2010).

There were two key concerns regarding this particular piece of research. First the unethical recruitment and use of the research participants, in this case children who already had significant health problems. Second was the issue that the research evidence was incorrect. In this case, Wakefield could be accused of nonmaleficence in the sense that he did not meet, at the very least, the first and second criteria highlighted by Beauchamp and Childress, that of not inflicting evil or harm and preventing evil or harm.

It is estimated that three million children aged between 18 months to 18 years have missed either their first or second MMR vaccination in the UK and there has consequently been a dramatic rise in the number of cases of measles in England and Wales in recent years. Primary Care Trusts have been provided with additional funds, particularly in London where vaccination rates are at the lowest, to run MMR catch-up programmes.

The principles of nonmaleficence

As we have seen the obligation of nonmaleficence is not only to not inflict harm but also to not "impose risks of harm". An individual can cause harm or place another person at risk of harm without malicious intent. This represents the principle of due care and determines whether an individual was taking sufficient and appropriate care to avoid causing harm.

For a legal case example, see: *Smith v Leech Brain Co* (1962)

In some emergency pre-hospital scenarios, practitioners can often impose risks of harm upon themselves.

Negligence

In essence, negligence is the absence of due care. Within the healthcare profession, negligence usually involves departure from specific standards that govern care. Negligence refers to two types of scenario: first the intention of unreasonable risks of harm, and second the unintentional imposition of harm. In the first scenario the practitioner knowingly inflicts an unwarranted risk – such as failing to provide antibiotic therapy to a patient with an obviously infected wound. In the second scenario, the practitioner unknowingly inflicts a harmful act that s/he should have known to avoid. An example would be leaving a patient's notes clearly visible for others to read.

Although in both scenarios the practitioner is to blame, the level of blame will vary depending on the context. In legal terms, practice that falls below a specified, accepted standard of due care will be the benchmark by which responsibility is measured. The moral responsibility for harm sometimes caused through healthcare practice consists of the following four duty of care elements. For harm to occur:

- The professional must have a duty to the affected party.
- The professional must breach that duty.
- The affected party must experience harm.
- The harm must be caused by the breach of duty.

Professional malpractice caused by negligence involves not following professional standards of care. The regulatory bodies of the Health Professions Council (HPC), the NMC and the professional body of the College of Paramedics/British Paramedics Association set out their standards for practice to which professionals are required to adhere (HPC, 2008; NMC, 2008b; College of Paramedics/British Paramedic Association, 2008).

Claims for negligence

Negligence can be defined as "actionable harm". NHS negligence claims have a potential value of some £4 billion. Between 2004 and 2005, 5609 claims of clinical negligence and 3766 claims of non-clinical negligence were brought against the NHS (NHSLA, 2009). Almost £503 million was paid out in connection with clinical negligence claims in 2004–2005 and an analysis of all clinical claims handled by the NHSLA since its inception in 1995 revealed that:

- 38.01% were abandoned by the claimant
- 43.1% settled out of court
- 1.97% settled in court in favour of the patient
- 0.5% settled in court in favour of the NHS, and
- 16.42% remain outstanding.

Perhaps one of the best-documented, and much debated, cases in relation to negligence is the case of *Bolitho v City and Hackney Health Authority* (1997). This case involved airway management and although this occurred in a hospital setting, it could just as easily have occurred in the pre-hospital setting.

Patrick Bolitho, a two-year-old boy was admitted to St Bartholomew's Hospital, London with croup in January 1984. Following a short period of fluctuating respiratory status, Patrick suffered two episodes of acute respiratory distress, from which he recovered spontaneously. During these attacks, a senior doctor, summoned by the ward sister, failed to attend or send a deputy. Patrick subsequently suffered a cardiac arrest and despite attempts to resuscitate him, he suffered "catastrophic" brain damage and later died.

In this sad case, there were two legal issues to consider. The first was the doctor's failure to attend Patrick. It was generally accepted that there was a breach of duty by the senior doctor in failing to attend Patrick when summoned, or arranging for someone else to do so. The second issue was the dispute over Patrick's treatment. The judge felt that a competent doctor would have assessed Patrick and performed an endotracheal intubation earlier in the afternoon following the second episode of respiratory distress. A total of eight experts were summoned to the court by the prosecution and they all agreed that any "competent" doctor would have intubated Patrick after the second episode. The defence called three expert clinicians, all of whom, relying on the ward sister's account, stated that it would not have been appropriate to intubate Patrick.

The judge took into account both of the opposing expert clinicians' views, concluding that if the senior doctor had attended and not intubated Patrick, she would have met the accepted level of skills and competence, and therefore decided that there had been no breach of duty of care on her part, and that this had not contributed to Patrick's death.

In the Bolitho case, the Judge's rationale was based on the case of *Maynard v West Midlands Regional Health Authority* (1985) in which the judge's preference for one body of expert opinion over another is not sufficient to establish negligence in a practitioner whose actions had been deemed competent by experts in the same field.

In medicine, negligence cannot be established by preferring one expert opinion to another. At the Court of Appeal, the Bolitho case was dismissed, referring to the Bolam Test, quoting that a doctor was not guilty of negligence if s/he acted in accordance with the "practice accepted as proper by a responsible body of medical men skilled in that particular art". The argument was first, that the Bolam Test was not applicable in this case since the question was not specifically about the level of care provided but rather whether the doctor failing to attend Patrick was the cause of his condition and subsequent death. Second, Patrick's family argued that the judge in the original case had misdirected himself by treating this as being the most relevant aspect in the case.

Managing emergencies

An exception to the above principle is that of a doctor who will be judged according to the standard of a reasonably experienced doctor in the emergency care field. In relation to treatment decisions taken in an emergency, a doctor will not be found negligent simply because a reasonably competent doctor would have made a different decision, given more time and information.

This principle was highlighted in the case of *Hotson v East Berkshire Area Health Authority* (1987) and focused on the nature of causation. It discarded the idea that patients can sue their doctors for the loss of a chance to get better, when doctors fail to do as good a job as they could have done in an emergency situation. The case was that of a 13-year-old boy who fell 12ft from a tree sustaining a traumatic fracture of the left femoral epiphysis. On examination at the hospital, the fracture was missed; the correct diagnosis not made until five days later when he was diagnosed with avascular necrosis. The condition was serious and by the time the claimant was 20 years of age, he was suffering from a deformity of his hip joint, which was restricting his mobility and causing permanent disability.

The judge ruled that even if the correct diagnosis had been reached at the initial presentation, there was still a 75% risk of him developing his disability. However the doctor's breach of duty had turned that risk into inevitability, thereby denying the claimant a 25% chance of a good recovery. Damages awarded included £11 500, representing 25% of the full value of the damages awardable for the claimant's disability. At the subsequent Appeal, the question was whether his injury was caused by the fall or by the health authority's negligence in delaying treatment. It was decided that as the fall had caused the injury, negligence on the part of the health authority was irrelevant in regard to the claimant's disability. The judge concluded that had the correct diagnosis and treatment been instigated initially, this would not have prevented his disability and therefore the claimant had failed on the issue of causation. It was therefore irrelevant to consider the question of further damages.

Clinical guidelines

Clinical guidelines are an accepted aspect of every practitioner's clinical life. The vast majority are based upon evidence-based research and are becoming increasingly relied upon in legal cases of clinical negligence. Guidelines are now the preferred term since the use of the term protocol was discouraged by the former NHS Executive due to its directive nature.

As clinical guidelines are being increasingly used in evidence, it is crucial that someone in authority compiles them (usually a team or panel of relevant experts), that they are clearly stated, in context, and it is obvious to whom they apply.

In another example, the case of *Early v Newham Health Authority* (1994) concerned a 13-year-old girl who recovered consciousness while still paralysed following an unsuccessful attempt to intubate her in preparation for an appendectomy. She panicked and was in great distress until she had recovered. The anaesthetic Senior House Officer had correctly followed the health authority's Failed Intubation Procedure, which had been written in conjunction with the health authority's eight consultant anaesthetists. The girl sued the health authority, claiming that the SHO was incompetent and negligent and that the Failed Intubation Procedure he followed was faulty and flawed. Her claim failed and, after applying a risk–benefit analysis, Deputy Judge Bennett QC concluded that the small risk of transient consciousness was far outweighed by the avoidance of the far greater risk of injury due to hypoxia – as in line with nonmaleficence. It could not be said that the guidelines were such that no reasonably competent authority would have adopted them.

NICE guidelines

The NICE guidelines are now an everyday aspect of clinical life, being widely disseminated and implemented. The Commission for Health Improvement, as the independent regulator of NHS performance, has the powers to monitor and ensure implementation of the NICE guidelines. Such guidelines will be authoritative, forming a new "normative" framework for the evidence of the standard of care to which doctors are required to conform. Professor Sir Michael Rawlins, the Chairman of NICE, is reported to have stated that "NICE guidelines are likely to constitute a reasonable body of opinion for the purposes of litigation. Doctors are advised to record their reasons for deviating from guidelines; deviation may not be regarded as logically defensible...".

Of course the NICE guidelines apply to a wide range of healthcare professionals, not just doctors, who will presumably fall into the group to which Professor Rawlins refers. In healthcare, it needs to be established that the act or omission caused the alleged damage and was reasonably foreseeable.

Another relevant case is that of *Barnett v Chelsea and Kensington Hospital Management Committee* (1968).

Beneficence

The principle of beneficence refers to the moral obligation to act for the benefit of others. As stated earlier Frankena (1973), cited in Beauchamp and Childress (2009), divided the principle of beneficence into the four general obligations of not inflicting, preventing and removing evil or harm, and promoting good.

The first obligation of not inflicting evil or harm refers to nonmaleficence; the remaining three obligations refer to beneficence, as stated earlier. These three latter obligations require a helping action of some kind and as such form the basis of beneficence. There are two aspects of beneficence: positive beneficence and utility. Positive beneficence requires an individual to provide a benefit to others whereas utility requires an individual to balance the benefits, risks and costs to produce the best overall effect.

The ethical principle of utilitarianism, sometimes referred to as utility, is based on the concept of beneficence. Some ethicists believe that beneficence is not obligatory but is an optional act. However the line between an obligation

Table 8.4. Differences between the rules of beneficence and nonmaleficence	
Nonmaleficence	*Beneficence*
Negative prohibition of actions	Present positive requirements of action
Must be followed impartially	Need not be followed impartially
Provide moral rationale for legal prohibitions of some forms of conduct	Generally do not provide reasons for legal punishment when an individual fails to abide by rules
	Adapted from Beauchamp and Childress (2009)

(such as rescuing a drowning person) and an ideal (such as donating to charity) are blurred in beneficence, but the two are distinct.

Beauchamp and Childress (2009) listed the five rules of beneficence:

- Protect and defend the rights of others.
- Prevent harm from occurring to others.
- Remove conditions that will cause harm to others.
- Help persons with disabilities.
- Rescue persons in danger.

The differences between beneficence and nonmaleficence are listed in *Table 8.4* and will be explored in some detail.

The second of Beauchamp and Childress' rules, "prevent harm from occurring to others" is based on being morally prohibited from causing harm to another individual although we are morally permitted to assist those with whom we have a special relationship, such as a patient, since we have entered into an agreed relationship with the patient as their practitioner. We are obligated to act nonmaleficently to everyone at all times (i.e. we generally do not stab or wound others) but it is not possible to act beneficently towards all people (i.e. donate money to every charity). It can be concluded that we are obliged to follow some rules of beneficence impartially – we can rescue that drowning man if we deem ourselves good swimmers and there is, therefore, relatively little personal risk.

There is also a distinction between specific and general beneficence, sometimes referred to as obligatory and nonobligatory beneficence. Specific beneficence, as the name suggests, is aimed at specific groups, such as children, friends, and families. General beneficence is aimed at others, or general groups, beyond these relationships. Most of us would agree that we would help or assist our own children, friends or families if required. However the concept of general or nonobligatory beneficence is less clear.

These obligations, by definition, relate to helping or assisting people we do not know or whose values are unknown to us. We are not able to help everyone, and to assist those unknown to us around the world in need of the basic requirements of life after natural disasters, such as earthquakes, would place significant demands on our beneficence. Some paramedics and nurses belong to volunteer international search and rescue teams, giving their free time to assist others in dire need. This extreme form of beneficence can cause harm to these volunteering individuals, such as injuries or risk of infection, and causes serious disruption to everyday life. This is a moral ideal and, whilst highly commendable, is not an obligation.

As the term beneficence generally refers to actions that promote the well-being of others, this means taking actions that serve the best interests of our patients. Beauchamp and Childress (2009) identify beneficence as one of the core values of healthcare ethics although some scholars argue that beneficence is the only fundamental ethical principle. However the concept of autonomy can come into conflict with beneficence when a patient disagrees with the recommendations of a practitioner, whose suggestions are made in the patient's best interests. As practitioners, we may believe that it is in the best interest of the patient to cease some health-limiting activity such as smoking, illicit drug taking or excessive alcohol consumption. In the UK, as with most Western societies, the patient's autonomy will take precedence if he or she is deemed mentally competent and the patient's wishes, perhaps to refuse treatment and our sage advice, must be respected.

The management of pain

Since the overall established aim of healthcare is "to do good", one of the priority issues in the urgent care setting is that of pain management. This ranges from treating patients suffering acute pain from illness, such as myocardial infarction; or injury, such as major trauma; to managing exacerbations of pain in palliative and end-of-life care.

For many years paramedics have been somewhat the envy of their allied health colleagues in having the ability to administer a wide range of opiate medications. These have included morphine sulphate in moderate to severe pain in cardiac conditions and entonox in moderate to severe labour pain. However the identification, assessment and management of acute pain is often poor, even in hospital settings. Most clinical guidelines for pain management refer to the World Health Organisation Pain Relief Ladder that was initially developed for managing cancer pain (WHO, 2010). *Figure 8.2* outlines this management plan that is arguably applicable to all types of pain presenting in an urgent care setting.

Pain management guidelines

Unfortunately the current JRCALC Clinical Guidelines make no reference

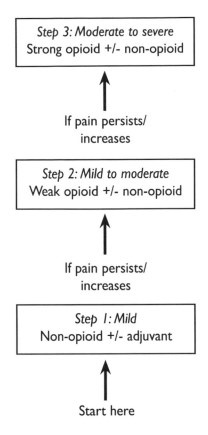

Figure 8.2. World Health Organisation Pain Relief Ladder.

to the WHO Pain Relief Ladder and although the theory of pain physiology and management is included in various paramedic training and education programmes, the depth of the subject varies considerably (JRCALC, 2006c). Most non-medical prescribing practitioners are able to administer or prescribe non-opioid pain relief, such as paracetamol and non-steroidal anti-inflammatory drugs, including aspirin or ibuprofen, and mild opioids, such as codeine. The stronger opioids such as morphine, either intravenous or oral, are available for administration by paramedics. Paramedics are currently unable to undertake non-medical prescribing programmes (although this position is currently under review) but those who have undertaken an academic paramedic practitioner programme, for example, will have the ability to prescribe a range of analgesics against Patient Group Directives.

NICE do not currently compile any clinical guidance on the management of acute pain. However, they do list a range of documentation to which practitioners are referred, such as the Australian and New Zealand College of Anaesthetists Guide, which helpfully refers to pre-hospital medicine (Macintyre et al, 2010).

The College of Emergency Medicine (2010) has published guidelines for the management of pain in adults and children. They largely reflect the WHO's Pain Relief Ladder, although opioids are not introduced until Step 3. The Royal College of Anaesthetists and the Pain Society's guidelines on pain management state that "the relief of pain should be a fundamental objective of any health service' (Royal College of Anaesthetists and the Pain Society, 2003: 1). Similarly, the *Taking Healthcare to the Patient: Transforming NHS Ambulance Services* document recommended that "pain should be better assessed and pain relief more widely used, particularly with children" (Department of Health, 2005c: 59).

The terminology is interesting, as most palliative approaches would recommend using the term pain control as opposed to pain relief. However the latter is arguably more achievable in the urgent and pre-hospital care scenario, where the immediate relief of acute pain is urgently required and is often the reason for calling the ambulance service or visiting an emergency department.

Paramedic pain management

Despite the ability of the paramedic to administer the strongest of opioid analgesics, as a professional group, their traditional training falls woefully short on the supporting pathophysiology, pharmacology and management of acute pain. This valuable knowledge is now delivered through some of the higher education institution education programmes. Giordano (2009) argued that if the management of pain were to be authentic for practitioners it requires knowledge of both the pathology of pain and the available treatments. The basic principles of pharmacology, such as pharmacodynamics and pharmacokinetics, are also required to ensure the practitioner has a holistic understanding of the principles and physiology of pain.

In addition, the academic preparation of practitioners in prescribing aids the decision making process in advanced practice. The concern for many practitioners working in urgent or pre-hospital care is when do the risks of administering opioid analgesia outweigh the benefits and who should make that decision, in other words, to act beneficently? The majority of urgent care practitioners are not pain specialists, yet they are presented with patients in acute pain on a daily basis, and with the lack of appropriate training, this pain is commonly undertreated and effective treatment often delayed (College of Emergency Medicine, 2010).

Central to pain management guidance is the need to respect every patient and to listen and value their reports regarding the nature and severity of pain. The JRCALC guidance on pain assessment refers to patients suffering pain from unusual sources, such as severe pruritus and dyspnoea. These patients can be in considerable pain even if perhaps not appearing, on initial assessment, to be in need of analgesia. Practitioners often feel frustrated and concerned if patients report unrelieved pain and there is an apparent tendency to avoid prescribing opiates stemming from a misguided fear of dependency and abuse (Macpherson, 2009).

This discomfort in prescribing or administering opiate analgesia impacts greatly on the patient, and practitioners may forget to consider how this affects patient's lives. To act beneficently or "to do good" as practitioners, we need to recognise our own failings or perhaps lack of education and call upon pain specialist colleagues when initial attempts at pain management are unsuccessful. Macpherson (2009) argued that, to be an "ethical practitioner", we need to learn about and understand pain, to follow pain guidelines and consult with pain specialists when our initial efforts fail, rather than labelling patients as hypochondriacs or drug seekers. Patients may indeed fall into the latter two categories, however this does not necessarily mean they are not in pain when they fracture their femur. More emphasis needs to be placed on examining our own beliefs and values in relation to pain and pain management.

Having an understanding of the knowledge, skill, attitudes and behaviours that are required for ethical practice, in respect of a patient's autonomy and beneficence, are essential, but are often missing from the paramedic training curriculum. Failing to understand our own attitudes and beliefs can potentially lead us to violate the ethical rights of our patients by undertreating pain. Some practitioners, and doctors are included here, misinterpret patient autonomy in pain management by withholding opiates, against guideline advice, perhaps by imposing their own experiences and attitudes towards pain, onto the patient.

Dignity

Goldenberg (2009) argued that all practitioners justify their role in relation to the ethical principles of autonomy, nonmaleficence, beneficence and justice, but proposed a further principle was required; that of dignity. The act of being beneficent or "doing good unto others" in the clinical context often means taking actions to serve the best interests of the patient although, as we have seen, there may be a disagreement as to what actually constitutes the best interests of the patient.

Goldenberg (2009) also suggested that dignity was the right of both the patient and the practitioner, with patients having the right to modesty and sympathy when they are suffering. Patients expect to be treated with respect, they do not expect the practitioner to be rude or make jokes or comments regarding their weight, personal hygiene or attire. The expectation of a professional and caring approach by the practitioner, with some regard to their illness is de rigueur. Similarly, the practitioner will expect courtesy and politeness from patients, even if they do not receive the treatment they anticipated.

Do we, and indeed can we, in an urgent care setting, always preserve the dignity of our patients? Clothes are frequently removed for clinical assessment and treatment but do we always ensure that we cover our patients adequately to ensure their dignity when we leave them to check results and summon additional help? The curtains in the emergency department and other clinics are neither soundproof nor sufficiently opaque to ensure privacy and confidentiality. Since there are often large numbers of clinical and hospital staff, visitors, relatives, police and other emergency services milling around in what are often very busy departments, the sight of some poor elderly patient, lying half dressed on a hospital trolley having just suffered a stroke suggests a lack of the most basic care.

The RCN launched the National Dignity Campaign in 2008, with principles that had been developed by the RCN's Emergency Care Association and the Patient's Association. The campaign's aim to was to make a visit to the emergency department less alarming for patients and to set out basic standards of care for trusts. The Campaign focused on areas such as the reception staff being welcoming, providing an estimate of how long patients could anticipate waiting, and obtaining the patient's informed consent for treatment. The RCN (2008) reported that many nurses completed their shift in the emergency department frustrated at their inability to provide compassionate, dignified care due to time constraints and targets. It seems almost unbelievable, in what is deemed a civilised, democratic society, that we require a major pharmaceutical company (the report was financially supported by Smith and Nephew) to fund a campaign highlighting what should be every patient's right and every practitioner's first act of caring.

Chochinov (2007) reported that patients who were not being treated with dignity were in a position of what he termed "acquired vulnerability". Although the concept of dignity stems initially from palliative care, there is no reason why patients, regardless of their condition, should not be treated with dignity. Chochinov proposed an ABCD checklist that should be fundamental in ensuring dignity. The mnemonic represented a core framework of Attitudes, Behaviour, Compassion and Dialogue, and is outlined in *Table 8.5*. Chochinov argued that this framework was easy to remember, empirically based and would assist in restoring the dignity of patients wherever they were in the healthcare system.

Justice

Justice is based on what is morally right, and is considered the fourth ethical principle. Fair, appropriate and equitable access to treatment could be defined as justice in biomedical ethics. Justice is difficult to quantify since it has different meanings for different people but its basic tenet is that of fairness.

Table 8.5. The Dignity ABCD Framework

Attitude

• How would I feel in this patient's situation? • What is leading me to this conclusion? • Are my assumptions accurate?	• Make an effort to make these questions a part of your reflective practice • Consider undertaking some continuing professional development or furthering your knowledge in challenging some of your attitudes and assumptions if they are affecting patient care

Behaviour

• Always ask patients for permission before you perform a clinical examination (routine for you but not for the patient) • Limit your conversation until the patient is completely dressed/covered • Demonstrate to the patient that they have your full attention	• Present information in a language the patient can understand • Maintain eye contact and keep at a comfortable level to communicate with the patient • Information about a major health issue can be overwhelming – be prepared to present the information several times

Compassion

• Watch films, read novels, go to the theatre and observe other portrayals of the human condition – there is a world outside clinical medicine • Listen and consider personal stories that surround the illness • Demonstrate empathy	• If and where applicable, use touch to convey compassion • Try to acknowledge people beyond their illness • Attempt to identify with those that are suffering

Dialogue

• Communicate – "I can only imagine what you are going through" (may sound trite but means a great deal to the patient) • Consider: What should I know about this person to help me take the best care of them? • Who could be here to support you?	• Make some referrals – consider who else could be involved at this point • Who else will be affected by this change in health?

Adapted from Chochinov (2007)

Justice in healthcare is debated due to the ever-increasing requirements for healthcare against access to diminishing resources, which challenges even the most prudent of healthcare providers.

Distributive justice refers to the distribution of rights in society and is distinguished from other types of justice, such as criminal justice. Beauchamp and Childress (2009: 241) refer to it as "fair, equitable and appropriate distribution determined by justified norms that structure the terms of social cooperation". A number of theories relate to distributive justice, such as egalitarian or utilitarian theory. Generally in distributive theories, the manner in which the goods are delivered is not due to any form of coercion or force. Any theories of distributive justice need to address three questions:

- What are the "goods" to be distributed – are they healthcare, wealth, power, etc., or a combination of these?
- Who will receive these "goods"?
- How will these "goods" be distributed – will it be based on need, being equal, etc?

The utilitarian principle is of the "greatest happiness for the greatest number of people" as identified by philosopher John Stuart Mill (Mill, 1962). Egalitarianism is discussed below.

Egalitarianism

Egalitarianism was defined by American philosopher John Rawls (1921–2002) and challenged other distributive justice theories of the day. In egalitarianism "goods" (healthcare in this context) are distributed equally. Rawls often referred to egalitarianism as "justice as fairness". Rawls' view was that these principles offered individuals the middle ground between altruism (selfless concern for the welfare of others, e.g. Mother Teresa) and egotism (enhancing favourable views of oneself). Humans on the whole are reasonable and rational beings, in that they are usually happy to achieve such ends together if they have mutually acceptable regulating principles.

In practice though, individuals have varying needs and aspirations, so finding a principle that suits everyone would be demanding. Rawls believed that this was a principle of equal basic liberties and his theory of egalitarianism had two conditions – the first that every individual is permitted the maximum of basic liberty and second, that once this liberty is assured, any inequalities, such as in social status, income, etc., are to be allowed. Although Rawls did not discuss his theory in relation to health, his philosophy has been applied to healthcare institutions, which would only work if they met the two stipulations. This positive societal obligation, in which any barriers were removed, would therefore ensure that any healthcare institution met all individuals' basic needs, regardless of income, wealth and status. This is essentially the intended basis to the NHS of course.

Distributive justice in action

In the UK, the principle of justice is perhaps best highlighted with regard to clinical guidelines. Whilst this might not initially appear to be an obvious choice, the NICE guidelines have been viewed as a form of rationing by some, with complaints and criticisms regarding the availability of treatment, termed the "postcode lottery" by a number of authors. Leaman argues that the NICE guidance is now "dictating standard medical practice" (Leaman, 2009: 627) and the guidance is flawed, being the opinion of an expert academic panel when little evidence exists. However the biggest challenge is that such guidance is being increasingly used in legal cases, with lawyers questioning practitioners why such guidelines have not been rigorously adhered to. This misses the entire point, since guidelines are just that – to act as guide for practice – with the JRCALC guidance being a prime example of guidelines that are advisory and developed to assist practitioners (Gregory, 2010).

The Bolam Test and the Bolitho case highlighted earlier, were cases where the judge accepted the opinions of the medical experts. However this was later challenged in *Marriott v West Midlands Regional Health Authority* (1999), a rare example where the courts deemed that the expert medical opinion did not support the case.

The Marriott case centred on a male patient who fell and was rendered unconscious. He remained unconsciousness for 30 minutes and was admitted to hospital for observation and investigation. Following his discharge the next day, he began to suffer from headaches, anorexia and lethargy. Eight days after the fall he contacted his GP who, having assessed him at home and finding no abnormality, recommended the patient remain at home, use analgesia and contact the GP again if his condition deteriorated. Four days later, the patient's condition had significantly deteriorated and he was re-admitted to hospital for surgery to remove an extradural haemorrhage and treatment for a skull fracture. Following surgery, the patient was left paralysed with a speech disorder. The patient subsequently sued the hospital for negligence, claiming he was discharged too soon on the first occasion and that his GP was negligent for not referring him back to the hospital sooner, maintaining that the GP should have realised the seriousness of his head injury.

The question of whether or not the GP was negligent for not undertaking a more thorough neurological examination and establishing the full extent of the patient's injury was considered. The expert witness for the patient claimed that given the length of time that Mr Marriott was unconscious, and the fact that his condition had not improved following discharge, should have alerted the GP to his need for immediate referral back to hospital. However the defendant's witness stated that given the small risk of extradural injury, the GP acted correctly. At Appeal, the case was upheld and the judge stated that, given the availability of neurological assessment at the local hospital and the considerable damage caused by the lesion which was avoidable, the GP was negligent. This case represented a sea change in medical negligence, given that both expert witnesses focused on the individual (i.e. the patient) rather than what would be considered reasonable practice (Brazier and Miola, 2000).

Samanta et al (2006) argued that some clinical guidelines impede clinical discretion and autonomy and are inflexible in clinical practice. The authors argued that clinical guidelines should not be taken as a *de facto* legal standard. The actual role of clinical guidelines in deciding legal standards of care is unclear with little evidence on the use of guidelines in clinical litigation in England and Wales. Baines (2005), for example, questioned the validity of the NICE head injury guidelines in clinical practice, arguing that the guidance, despite being a publication of a statutory authority, fell short. In a survey of the legal community, Samanta et al discovered that the legal profession referred to both NICE and Royal College guidelines in their clinical negligence cases.

A no-fault system was proposed in the *Making Amends* document (Department of Health, 2003a), although this was later rejected by the Chief Medical Officer due to the potential rise in claims. Although the Chief Medical Officer suggested that a fairer test than the Bolam Test was required, it was not included in the NHS Redress Bill, so the current test for redress remains the "avoidability test"– whereby an adverse event would be compensatable except when it results in an unavoidable complication, regardless of the treatment. Such proposals for reform are likely to resurface in the future as the Bolam standard evolves into one with greater reliance on guidelines.

The English courts do not uncritically accept guidelines as evidence of responsible or acceptable clinical practice. Since the author of clinical guidelines is rarely available to provide oral testimony in court, any such evidence is hearsay. Evidence of accepted clinical practice is usually introduced via an appropriate expert who is able to comment on practice and relevant literature, such as guidelines, to further support his or her opinion. Such opinion and application of these guidelines can be challenged further under cross-examination, regardless of whether or not they are mandatory.

For a legal case example, see:
Thomson v Blake-James & Others (1998)
Case involving measles vaccination where GP was found to be negligent in the case of a child who suffered a suspected seizure

Hucks v Cole (1968)
A case where a doctor failed to prescribe penicillin to a patient suffering from a septic skin condition

NICE guidelines and the rationing of healthcare

Allocating, or rationing, of healthcare is a fact of life. Since the inception of NICE in 1999 evidence-based clinical guidelines have advised some restrictions of certain therapeutic interventions. One such area is the management of low back pain, a commonly presenting symptom in urgent care and one for which NICE has published guidance (NICE, 2009b). Some critics argue that the NICE guidance is not evidence based, that it recommends treatments at an "arbitrary" rate and that the guideline development committee for back pain did not include a pain physician (Bartley, 2009; Munglani, 2009).The British Pain Society voted its president, Professor Paul Watson, out of office as some of its members disagreed with his support of the guidance. NICE was "outraged" and two eminent clinicians deemed this "professional victimisation at its worst'" and suggested that the Society did not accept evidence-based medicine (Rawlins and Littlejohns, 2009: 3028).

NICE's head injury guidelines caused similar issues (NICE, 2007). The guidelines recommended that patients presenting with a serious head injury, with a Glasgow Coma Score of less that 13 on initial assessment in the emergency department within a short post-injury time-frame, or with associated symptoms, should receive a computerised tomography (CT) scan within one hour. NICE's guidance suggested that the CT scan should replace the traditional skull x-ray in head injury management since its sensitivity is close to 100%. This represented a significant additional cost to the hospital, not to mention increased radiation exposure for the patients (Qureshi et al, 2005; Shavrat et al, 2006).

Much of the criticism surrounded the issue of why the early management of patients with head injuries required altering in the first place, since comparatively very few of the head injuries presenting to an emergency department required CT scans (Dunning and Lecky, 2004). The early head injury guidelines published by the Scottish Intercollegiate Guidelines Network (SIGN, 2000) in conjunction with the Royal College of Physicians in 2000 and the 1999 Report of the Working Party on the Management of Patients with Head Injuries published by the Royal College of Surgeons (RCS, 1999) in England used the skull x-ray for either determining admission to hospital for further observation or for CT scan. This was a poor test, as 25–50% of all patients attending with a minor head injury would require a skull x-ray, with 98% of patients having no fracture. Of the remaining 2% of patients, approximately 1 in 30 would be suffering from an underlying traumatic brain injury such as an intracranial haematoma that required surgical intervention.

The concern was that a large percentage of head-injured patients had traumatic brain injury with no fracture. CT is a highly sensitive test for traumatic brain injury when contrasted with skull x-ray. The RCS and SIGN guidelines were consensus documents and were not evidence-based and therefore could not be relied upon.

Summary

This chapter has focused on the importance of remembering that the first duty of medicine (and healthcare in general) is that the patient remains at the centre of care. Whilst this is undoubtedly implicit in the majority of literature, policy documents, White papers and so on, there is a tendency to "forget" or to overlook the fact that we are all here to care for patients. Occasionally we are patients ourselves and it is often this very experience that shapes our own attitudes and beliefs. In this regard, Pellegrino provided some helpful insights. According to Pellegrino, medical ethics is grounded in the patient–doctor relationship; that is to say in the philosophy of medicine, which is based on three tenets: first that illness and disease diminishes the integrity of human nature, changes self-image and limits freedom in many ways; second that the doctor or other healthcare professional promises to aid us when we are ill; and third that the technical aspects of care are undertaken with a morally correct decision that best serves the needs of the patient (Pellegrino, 1981).

References

Ayatollahi H, Bath PA, Goodacre S (2009) Accessibility versus confidentiality of information in the emergency department. *Emergency Medicine Journal* **26**(12): 857–60

Baines P (2005) NICE head injury guidelines: A review of the legal mandate. *Emergency Medicine Journal* **22**(10): 706–9

Barnett v Chelsea & Kensington Hospital Management Committee (1968) 1 All ER 1068

Bartley R (2009) Wishful thinking? 28 May Letters. *British Medical Journal Rapid Response*

Beauchamp TL, Childress JF (2009) *Principles of biomedical ethics*. (6th edn) New York: Oxford University Press

Black C, Kaye JA, Jick H (2002) Relation of childhood gastrointestinal disorders to autism: Nested case-control study using data from the UK General Practice Research Database. *British Medical Journal* **325**: 419–21

Bolitho v City and Hackney Health Authority (1997) 4 All ER 771

Brazier M, Miola J (2000) Bye Bye Bolam. A medical litigation revolution? *Medical Law Review* **8**(1): 85–114

Chochinov H (2007) Dignity and the essence of medicine: The A B, C, and D of dignity conserving care. *British Medical Journal* **335**(7612): 184–7

College of Emergency Medicine (2004) *Guidelines for the management of pain in adults*. London: CEM

College of Paramedics and British Paramedic Association (2008) *Paramedic*

Curriculum Guidance and Competence Framework. (2nd edn)
Derbyshire: CoP

Council of Europe (1950) *European Convention on Human Rights*. Available
from: http://www.hri.org/docs/ECHR50.html

D v NSPCC (1978) http://www.tooks.co.uk/download/061011_Fact_Finding_
and_Disclosure_For_Family_Lawyers.pdf

Declaration of Helsinki (1996) *British Medical Journal* **313**(7070): 1448–9

Department of Health (1997) *The Caldicott Committee: Report on the review
of patient-identifiable information*. London: HMSO

Department of Health (2003a) *Making Amends: A consultation paper setting
out proposals for reforming the approach to clinical negligence in the
NHS*. London: HMSO

Department of Health (2003b) *Confidentiality. NHS Code of Practice*.
London. HMSO

Department of Health (2005c) *Taking healthcare to the patient: Transforming
NHS Ambulance Services*. London: HMSO

Dimond B (1993) Consent and the unconscious patient in the Accident and
Emergency department. *Accident and Emergency Nursing* **1**: 171–3

Dunning J, Lecky F (2004) The NICE guidelines in the real world: A practical perspective. *Emergency Medicine Journal* **21**(4): 404–7

Early v Newham Health Authority (1994) 5 Med LR 214

Etchells E (1996) *Bioethics for clinicians: 4. Voluntariness*. Canadian
Medical Association Journal **155**: 1083–6

Foëx BA (2001) The problem of informed consent in emergency medicine
research. *Emergency Medicine Journal* **18**(3): 198–204

Frampton A (2005) Reporting in gunshot wounds by doctors in emergency
department: A duty or a right? Some legal and ethical issues surrounding
breaking confidentiality. *Emergency Medicine Journal* **22**(2): 84–6

General Medical Council (2009) *Confidentiality: Reporting gunshot and knife
wounds*. London: GMC

General Medical Council (2010) *Dr Andrew Jeremy Wakefield. Determination
on Serious Professional Misconduct (SPM) and sanction*. London: GMC

Giordano J (2009) The neuroscience of pain, and neuroethics of pain care.
Neuroethics **3**(1): 89–94

Goldenberg S (2009) Medical ethics. *Journal of Continuing Education Topics
and Issues* **11**(2): 60–3

Gregory P (2010) JRCALC: Advice or requirement? (Editorial). *Journal of
Paramedic Practice* 2(1): 5

Health Professions Council (2007) *Standards of proficiency: Paramedics*.

London: HPC

Health Professions Council (2008) *Standards of conduct, performance and ethics*. London.

Hotson v East Berkshire Area Health Authority (1987) 2 All ER 909

Hucks v Cole (1968) http://www.publications.parliament.uk/pa/ld199798/ ldjudgmt/jd971113/boli02.htm Norrie, 1985

Hughes G (2009) Knife crime reporting. *Emergency Medicine Journal* **26**(2): 80

Joint Royal Colleges Ambulance Liaison Committee (JRCALC) (2006c) *Management of pain in adults*. Warwick: JRCALC

Joint Royal Colleges Ambulance Liaison Committee (JRCALC) and the Ambulance Service Association (ASA) (2006b) *UK Ambulance Service Clinical Practice Guidelines*. Warwick: JRCALC & ASA

Leaman A (2009) NICE: Mostly a bad idea. *Emergency Medicine Journal* **26**(9): 627–8

Loefler I (2002) Why the Hippocratic ideals are dead. *British Medical Journal* **324**(7351): 1463

Macintyre PE, Schug SA, Scott DA, Visser EJ, Walker SM (2010) *APM: SE Working Group of the Australian and New Zealand College of Anaesthetists and Faculty of Pain Medicine: Acute pain management: scientific evidence* (3rd edn). Melbourne: ANZCA and FPM

Macpherson C (2009) Undertreating pain violates ethical principles. *Journal of Medicl Ethics* **35**(10): 603–6

Malette v Shulman (1991) 2 Med LR 162

Marriott v West Midlands Regional Health Authority (1999) Lloyds Medical Reports 23

Maynard v West Midlands Regional Health Authority (1985) 1 All ER 635

Medical Protection Society (2008) *Consent – children and young people*. London: MPS

Munglani R (2009) NICE guideline on low back pain flawed. 31st May Letters. *British Medical Journal Rapid Response*

National Health Service Litigation Authority (NHSLA) (2009) *Reports and Accounts 2009*. London: NHSLA

NICE (National Institute for Health and Clinical Excellence) (2007) *Triage, assessment, investigation and early management of head injury in infants, children and adults*. London: National Collaborating Centre for Acute Care

NICE (National Institute for Health and Clinical Excellence) (2009b) *Low back pain. Early management of persistent non-specific low back pain*.

London: NICE

NMC (Nursing and Midwifery Council) (2008a) *Covert administration of medicines - disguising medicine in food and drink*. London: NMC.

NMC (Nursing & Midwifery Council) (2008b) *Code: Standards of conduct, performance and ethics for nurses and midwives*. London: NMC

OPSI (Office of Public Sector Information) (1967) *Public Health Act (Northern Ireland 1967)*. London: OPSI

OPSI (Office of Public Sector Information) (1984) *Public Health (Control of Disease) Act 1984*. London: OPSI

OPSI (Office of Public Sector Information) (1988) *Access to Health Records Act. 1988*. London: OPSI

OPSI (Office of Public Sector Information) (1998a) *Road Traffic Act 1998*. London: OPSI.

OPSI (Office of Public Sector Information) (1998b) *Public Health (Infectious Diseases) Regulations 1998*. London: OPSI

OPSI (Office of Public Sector Information) (1998c) *Data Protection Act [DPA] 1998*. London: OPSI

OPSI (Office of Public Sector Information) (2000a) *Access to Health Records Act (AHRA) 2000*. London: OPSI

OPSI (Office of Public Sector Information) (2000b) *Terrorism Act 2000*. London: OPSI

OPSI (Office of Public Sector Information) (2008) *Public Health etc (Scotland) Act 2008*. London: OPSI

Peate I, Potterton J (2009) Hush! Let's talk confidentiality. *British Journal of Healthcare Assistants* 3(12): 609–12

Pellegrino ED (1981) From medical ethics to a moral philosophy of the professions. In Walter JK, Klein EP (eds) *The story of bioethics*. Washington, DC: Georgetown University Press

Quality Assurance Agency for Higher Education (2001) *Nursing Benchmark statement: Health care programmes Phase 1*. Gloucester: QAA

Quality Assurance Agency for Higher Education (2004) *Paramedic science Benchmark statement: Health care programmes. Phase 2*. Gloucester: QAA

Qureshi AA, Mulleady V, Patel A, Porter KM (2005) Are we able to comply with NICE head injury guidelines? *Emergency Medicine Journal* 22(12): 861–2

Rawlins M, Littlejohns P (2009) NICE on back pain. NICE outraged by ousting of pain society president. *British Medical Journal* 339(7715): 3028

Rogers v Whitaker (1992) http://www.bioethics.org.au/Resources/Online%20

Articles/Opinion%20Pieces/0503%20Rogers%20v%20Whitaker%20 duty%20of%20disclosure.pdf

Royal College of Anaesthetists and the Pain Society (2003) *Pain management services. Good practice.* London: The Royal College of Anaesthetists and the Pain Society

Royal College of Nursing (2008) *RCN puts dignity at the heart of emergency care.* London: RCN

Royal College of Surgeons of England (1999) *Report of the Working Party on the Management of Patients with Head Injuries.* London: RCS

Samanta A, Mello MM, Foster C, Tingle J, Samanta J (2006) The role of clinical guidelines in medical negligence litigation: A shift from the Bolam standard? *Medical Law Review* **14**(3): 321–66

SIGN (Scottish Intercollegiate Guidelines Network) (2000) *Early management of patients with a head injury. A national clinical guideline.* Edinburgh: SIGN

Shavrat BP, Huseyin TS, Hynes KA (2006) NICE guideline for the management of head injury: An audit demonstrating its impact on a district general hospital, with a cost analysis for England and Wales. *Emergency Medicine Journal* **23**(2): 109–13

Smith CM (2005) Origin and uses of *primum non nocere* – Above all, do no harm. *Journal of Clinical Pharmacology* **45**: 371-377

Smith v Leech Brain Co (1962) http://www.e-lawresources.co.uk/forum/ viewtopic.php?f=76&t=288 Maynard v .West Midlands Regional Health Authority (1985)

Swindell JS (2009) Two Types of Autonomy. *American Journal of Bioethics – Neuroscience* **9**(1): 52

Thomson v Blake-James and others (1998) 5 Lloyd's Rep Med 187

Wakefield, AJ, Murch SH, Anthony A, Linnel J, Casson DM, Malik M, Berelowitz M, Dhillon AP, Thomson MA, Harvey P, Valentine A, Davies SE, Walker-Smith JA (1998) Ileal-lymphoid-nodular hyperplasia, non-specific colitis, and pervasive development disorder in children. *Lancet* 351(9103): 637–42

World Health Organisation (2010) *Pain relief ladder.* Geneva: WHO

World Medical Association (1964) *WMA Declaration of Helsinki. Ethical Principles for Medical Research Involving Human Subjects* (updated 59th WMA General Assembly, Seoul, October 2008)

Index